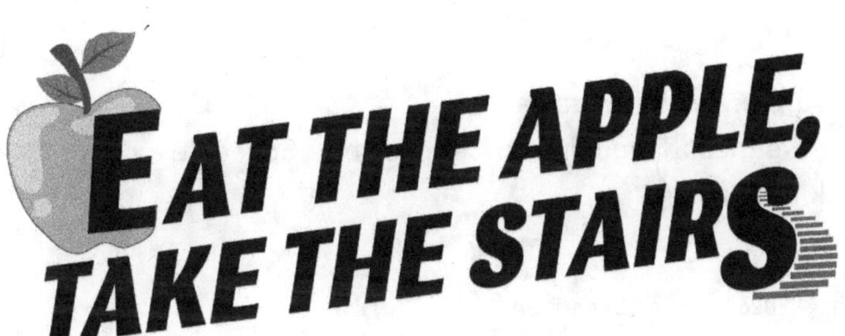

EAT THE APPLE, TAKE THE STAIRS

WEAVING WELLNESS THROUGH YOUR **"IMPOSSIBLE"** SCHEDULE

BY

DEREK OPPERMAN

Eat the Apple, Take the Stairs
Weaving Wellness Through Your "Impossible" Schedule
by Derek Opperman

ISBN: 979-8-234-00215-0

Edition: First Edition

Design and production: BGC LA

Editing: Derek Opperman, Nory Oakes and Morgan Ellis

Publisher: LifeUP Publishing

Website: www.lifeuphealthcoaching.com

Derek Opperman is a fifteen-time-certified trainer and integrative health coach, a Fortune 500 keynote speaker, and a corporate wellness program designer. He helps busy parents and professionals reclaim their energy, confidence, and long-term health with simple, sustainable strategies.

CONTENTS

INTRODUCTION

"You. You there. What did you just put in your pocket?"

I froze, as if I didn't hear the cop's words.

"Déjame verlo."

"Let me see it," the officer commanded, presenting one open hand in front of me, expecting suspected contraband... one hand on his gun.

A million thoughts swirled in my head at once.

Do I run? Do I fight? Do I make him search me?

Another officer flanked me and my friend. No running now.

I was fucked..

I slowly pulled out a bag of cocaine and handed it to him.

"Sabes que la posesión de cocaína es un delito que conlleva prisión, ¿verdad?"

My Spanish-speaking friend translated, but I got the gist without needing him to.

"My. Life. Is. Over." I thought.

I cannot go to jail. Let alone a Mexican jail. They'll eat me alive.

What's worse, I was in Mexico at this time to help run a health retreat! While out partying, I had a dozen students sleeping back at the resort expecting me to run a stretch and foam-rolling class with them the next morning.

I could see them talking now...

"Where's Derek?" they'd ask, as they realized I wasn't present at our community breakfast.

"Oh, he's uh... currently in jail on a cocaine possession charge," my co-facilitator would tell them.

I could hear their gasps of horror and judgment ringing in my ears already.

"What a piece of shit I am. Such a hypocrite. Holding the beacon of health high in one hand and a bag of illegal substance behind my ready-to-be-cuffed back in the other."

This was not supposed to be part of my story. Guys like me don't get in trouble like this.

Yet here I was, moments away from seeing the facade of immaculate health and mindfulness come crashing down.

"Derek... Derek... DEREK!" my friend said, slapping me back to reality.

"The cops want $500 and they said they'll let us walk. There's an ATM over there. I'll take the cash out. Let's get this over with."

My heart slowly drops back down to my chest after I see my friend pay off the cop in the near distance.

We walked, shaken but free men.

The crisis was averted, but shame remained intact.

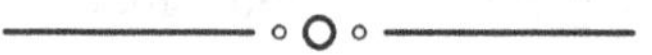

A smarter individual would've taken that lesson to the bank and cleaned up their act. Unfortunately, the near-miss in Mexico was just a blip on my rap sheet. Between 21 and 30 years old, I was well-versed in the Deadly Sins.

I was a goon, getting in fist fights at parties and outside nightclubs.

I was a substance abuser, spending a year's worth of college tuition on drugs and alcohol.

I was a deviant, questioned by authorities for public intoxication or driving under the influence on multiple occasions.

I was a glutton, ballooning up to 210 lbs on my typically 180 lb frame, eating everything in the name of "bulking."

In between having a taste for partying hard on the weekends, I was, (believe it or not), a "fitness professional" who had just opened his first gym with plans to open more.

I really could fool someone into thinking I had life and health all fig-ured out.

Weekdays I ate decently, worked out hard, trained and coached clients. By Friday night I was ready to break out and go wild. Parties. Nightclubs. Girls. Alcohol. Drugs. Late night fast food. Come Sunday morning, I was hungover and remorseful—hitting the farmers' market and church to repent.

Back on the straight and narrow... until Friday.

Rinse and repeat.

I knew it was hypocritical—miles away from the temperance and moderation I was preaching with clients. But hey, at least I was still "looking" the part—a true Dr. Jekyll and Mr. Hyde experience.

At some point my guardian angel got tired of seeing my sorry ass in this endless loop and handed me the ultimate reality check:

A few months after the incident in Mexico, I was going to unexpectedly become a father with a woman I had just started dating.

I was floored.

This was not part of my plan.

"Guys like me don't get in trouble like this."

My Hyde was exposed—there was no way to spin this now.

The news put me at a crossroads: I could walk away from the baby and keep living the life I had... or figure out how to show up and be the role model my daughter deserved.

I chose the latter.

But not without plenty of resistance from Mr. Hyde along the way...

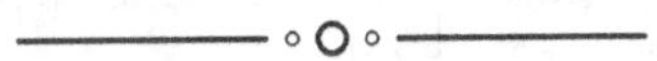

Having a newborn, a suddenly serious relationship, and opening a new business individually take loads of work—putting them all together at once left me spinning and overwhelmed. Being the sole breadwinner only intensified the pressure.

The role of responsible, mature Dr. Jekyll was a hard one to live up to all the time.

So, Hyde showed up again.

I acted out, drank, and did drugs to escape. Money was tight.

I withdrew emotionally. My girlfriend and I fought; my health suffered.

A year after my daughter was born I got caught publicly intoxicated and with drugs at a theme park.

I mean, a theme park?! C'mon man.

I got kicked out but luckily was not prosecuted. I was horribly embarrassed.

I was waiting for an Uber at the park exit with my now-fiancée.

"I still love you, but I think it's best you go home by yourself to think about this experience," she said.

That night, all alone, I couldn't stop looking at photos of my daughter.

Beautiful, sweet, smart, and innocent.

Those quiet hours forced me to confront the double life I was living.

"Is this the kind of role model you want to be for your daughter? What the hell are you running from? Is this life really so unbearable where you have to escape with alcohol and drugs?"

THE BOTTOM

Looking back on that evening, alone and depressed, I realized I had made up that my life was going to be over when the baby came—or at the very least, no longer under my control.

I thought showing up for my child had to mean there was no room for anything but work and parenting. No time for personal interests. No time for friends. No time for health.

I was convinced that letting go of the party life would leave me a one-dimensional suburban dad. Fat, stressed, sleep-deprived.

Even though I had no evidence of that being true, I had a really hard time surrendering that notion; the fear of that false reality became a trauma that took multiple run-ins with the law to slap me out of.

That night I learned that **anything great worth having is worth changing for.**

Booze and drugs couldn't be a part of my narrative going forward.

This wasn't a matter of sudden self-righteousness. It became a matter of leaving a legacy and being known for something beyond party stories and an eventual conviction.

So I committed.

I decided that night I was going to change—the life I truly wanted to live and be proud of depended on it.

So who am I to write a book about mindfulness, health and self-care for busy parents and professionals?

After all, I was none of those things at various stages of my life.

"Hypocrite... Imposter... Poser... Loser."

Yet the scars and warts I wear may be the perfect reason to write this book—not because of a pristine health track record, but because I've been in the mud and mire, succumbing to earthly desires and paying the price time and time again.

Through those breakdowns, I discovered, that every day brings the chance to choose something new. A new mindset, a new habit, a new way of being.

I had to get 100% responsible for the life I had up to this point and the one I actually wanted. I had to prioritize differently, because the small surplus of time I previously possessed was no longer available. If I was going to be a dad, a partner, a business person, and practice what I preached as a fitness professional, I was going to have to do life differently.

Up until then I partied, gorged, indulged, and abused my body.

I was going to have to level up to meet the newfound demands kids and career called for.

We don't need another Instagram prophet holding fitness commandments for all to behold. That was my old way—looking healthy while hiding the triple vodka and lime just out of frame.

But the pious life of a modern-day monk isn't realistic, either.

That dualistic thinking is what got me here in the first place.

We have to accept that perfection isn't going to happen all of the time.

Cheeseburgers taste good once in a while. A glass or two of wine shared with friends can be part of a life well-lived.

I had to integrate my Hyde a little bit so he shows up in controlled, moderate doses. On my terms. No more out-of-control bingeing on the weekends followed by shame-dieting during the week.

I needed help breaking out of that cycle.

I needed fresh perspective and small, manageable steps that had me feel like I was making progress without overwhelming my limited time and brain reserves.

I needed to find a way to weave wellness into my impossible schedule.

Through conscious self-discovery, behavior tracking, and emulating coaches and mentors, I started seeking out the best health practices that could fit into my already-full calendar.

"Working out for seven minutes is better than not working out at all."

"Eating protein and vegetables before starches helps curb blood sugar spikes."

"Drink water before coffee…"

"Get sunshine first thing in the morning…"

I was starting to see there was so much more to health than just hard workouts and eating fewer calories.

I realized I could feel great all week long—weekends included—by managing my environment and redefining relationships within my social circle. No FOMO. Just freedom.

I asked my party friends to get together with me earlier in the day for lunch or during the week for a workout so we could connect but not over late-night antics. I still had a burger and a beer on the weekends, but made sure to go for a walk after to help digestion.

I made wellness—comprehensive wellness—a game to play and to win.

THIS BOOK

The lessons in these pages were found through trial and error as a fallible partner, father, and fitness professional.

Some chapters were sourced the hard way—by learning from mistakes and making changes to avoid repeating that pain. Some I derived from learning through experts and mentors and experiencing those benefits firsthand.

Others were learned through the lens of clients, friends, and family who were also making their way through life—juggling kids, careers, setbacks and aiming to strike the perpetual balance of a healthy lifestyle through it all.

Each one of these stories is true. Names may change. Timelines may be condensed. But the stories are rooted in the real world by myself or people I know who have overcome health challenges and declared victory over past circumstances by making simple, conscious changes to their lifestyles.

I wrote this book alongside and to acknowledge my fellow moms and dads who didn't give up on their well-being in the face of daily challenges. Those who found a way to weave wellness through their "impossible" schedule—in hopes that you, dear reader, can do so as well.

Because life doesn't slow down. Time only speeds up as we grow older. And our health will forever remain a tertiary priority if we don't consciously choose otherwise—something to do when we "can get to it," "feel like it," or "when we're ready."

But that day may never come.

We're so prone to our habits that making sweeping lifestyle changes rarely stick long term—even if a windfall of time becomes available to practice them.

Instead, our best bet is to embody simple, manageable changes that fit into our lives right now. "Microshifts" that may seem small, otherwise inconsequential, yet are the basis for vibrant longevity.

The mission of this book is to bring healthy habits to the forefront of your mind by demonstrating where they can fit within your already

busy day—and the upside of employing them.

It's to support you to discover and weave wellness into your "impossible" schedule.

I share these practices because I do them to maintain my own health, despite a packed schedule and incessant temptations around me.

There is an access to become a little happier, healthier, and more connected in nearly every moment. We've just got to know where to look.

This book is best utilized experientially. I suggest you try on every chapter possible to see how it lands in your life—did it feel good, make sense, create value?

It's titled *"Eat the Apple, Take the Stairs"* for a reason!

Anything less than a hands-on experience will have these pages occur as "good to know" information and little more, leaving you with nothing but another book on the shelf and an opportunity missed.

When you employ and embody the practices within this book, you'll begin to discover that there's more time available to you than ever before. This book promotes efficiency and opportunity-seeking. To have you no longer ask, "What can I do?", but "How can I do it?"

When you apply that mindset to your health, it tends to spread to other people around you, too!

Partners will notice the difference in your waistline when they give you a squeeze. Co-workers will inquire about where you got all that energy and want in on it, too. Your kids will see and relate to you differently.

At some point during your transformation you may encounter resistance from some actors in your environment. We're all resistant to change initially—give them and yourself grace! Life is a long game. Remain steadfast in the pursuit of health and all will come around.

Heed my request now: make the changes small and make them consistently.

You'll discover it is the quality of actions, not quantity of actions that delivers a physical and mental transformation.

The Pareto Principle states that for many outcomes, roughly 80% of effects come from 20% of causes. Focus on the "vital few" that generate the majority of results rather than spreading efforts across the "trivial many."

So, release the belief that it takes hours of time in the gym and kitchen to get healthy again.

You wouldn't or couldn't do it that way regardless, would you?

We've got to take small, effective, repeatable steps that lead us to the desired outcomes.

Beginning something new requires a little faith in what cannot yet be seen. I will ask that you expand your vision and belief as to what's possible to achieve in a given day. Reaching our greater or greatest potential takes some suspension of limitations, and that takes some planning and consideration.

Expand your vision and beliefs, and you'll find yourself mastering health with more vibrant energy, time, and clarity than ever before.

Read on, see your own journey within the stories I share, and be inspired to think about what's possible with small, accessible changes.

HOW TO USE
THIS BOOK

> # No success is immediate. No collapse is sudden. They are both the result of the slight edge accruing momentum over time.
>
> - Jeff Olson

I've organized the habits in "flights" by order of difficulty to integrate into your busy life. The first few chapters are flights one, followed by flights two through seven.

My hope is that you'll begin with the easiest wellness "weaves" and score a few habit wins. Once you integrate these, begin expanding your vision of what true health for a busy person can look like by taking on the subsequent flights.

Of course, you may find you're already doing some of these actions—great for you! You may also find initial habits are more personally challenging than later ones. If you're one of those people who have to park as close to the store entrance as possible, getting extra steps in may be a particular obstacle!

All that to say, wellness is NOT a one-size-fits-all conversation. Observe these chapters accordingly.

Consider the process I offer as an ascension toward impactful habits from easiest to hardest (ish). Nothing is set in stone; see them as simply a means to effectively move through the book in a way I believe progresses one toward mastery little by little.

However you choose to play, just make sure to play.

Every time you implement one of these steps, you'll find yourself closer to developing hard-wired habits, having them eventually occur as an embodied part of you, not as something to cross off a checklist in order to achieve a temporary goal.

Welcome—I'm glad you're here. Let's begin.

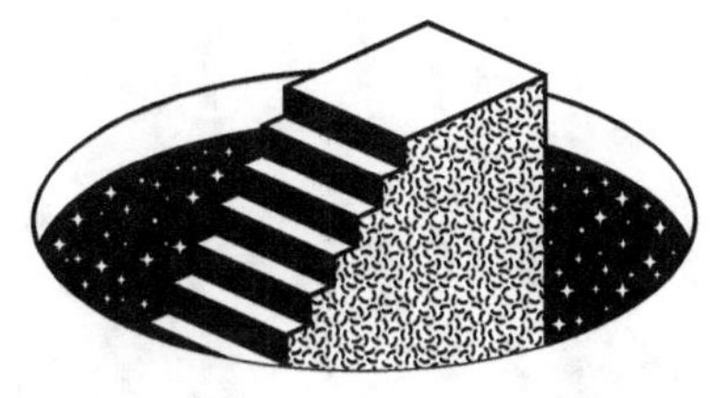

FIRST FLIGHT

Don't let "perfect" be the enemy of "done"

> # Le mieux est l'ennemi du bien.
>
> ## The best is the enemy of the good.
>
> - Voltaire

"Hey honey—how was your day?" I asked my then-fiancée, bopping into the house after a busy day of training clients (and not training myself).

Judging by the exhausted look on her face, it was harder than mine.

"Terrible. Sophie was up super early, and she wouldn't nap, so she was fussy and wouldn't let me put her down. I haven't gotten anything done!"

"Oye—sounds like a tough day, babe..."

"Yeah, I haven't started dinner and the house... ugh, this house!" she said, pointing around to the toys littered about our living room and dishes in the sink.

After another minute of venting, she composed herself a bit.

"Anyway—how are you? How was your day?"

"Good! Busy—full of clients and not much else but that..."

"Yeah?" she said, raising an eyebrow, suddenly aware there may be a request to field.

"Think I could have a quick workout?" I said quickly, grimacing and bracing for impact.

Her face went flat. Then silence. I smiled sheepishly.

"15 minutes. You've got 15 minutes."

"Thank you!"

I kissed her and ran out the door, knowing she may change her mind and that I didn't have a grace period.

I ran, nay, sprinted half a mile up the street to my in-law's condo complex gym (four minutes), did a circuit of pull-ups, shoulder presses, and v-up crunches twice through (seven minutes), and ran home (four minutes)—home in 15 to relieve my wife without feeling her wrath.

"Phew! Thanks, babe. Now, how can I help?"

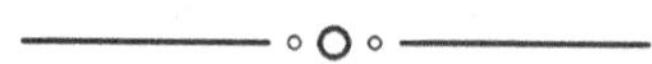

Stories like this one are often how my wife and I have made time for weaving wellness into our busy parenting and working lives.

If one or both of us are faced with a full day, we strive to create or negotiate a gap within a packed schedule... for a nap, for a mental health break in the sunshine, for a healthy snack, for a workout.

Was my 15-minute session record breaking by any means? Of course not. It was really just enough to work my lungs and muscles a bit, then head home to put my "father hat" on.

However, it was enough to do something positive and empowering for myself with the time I had available.

Sure, I could've just said, "Screw it, there's not enough time," or "Hopefully tomorrow will be better," or "We'll start fresh Monday," or "She sounds stressed, I better not ask."

Spoiler alert: If you're a parent, or working full-time (or both)—"start fresh Mondays" don't exist. Make the most of what you got when you've got it.

And you may be surprised that it's often more than enough!

It takes seven minutes for me to break a sweat at a moderate running pace.

It takes one to two sets of a strength-based exercise to build muscle (and neural connections to muscle) for untrained or minimally trained individuals.

Preparing a smoothie, snacks and a healthy lunch for tomorrow takes 8-15 minutes.

10-20-minute naps can be invigorating (I've taken a three-minute nap before—it can be done!).

We'd all love the time for a two-hour gym session, complete with a long stretch and sauna afterwards. Or nine hours of uninterrupted sleep. Or a half day to meal prep for the week.

But this book isn't for those people.

This book is for the mom of two who just dropped one kid off at school and has the other in a car seat behind her in the minivan, with a to-do list a mile long, but is tired of making excuses for why she can't cook healthy for herself or her family.

This book is for the dad with sales deadlines that have him in a pressure cooker who is looking for something other than drinking too much to cut the stress.

This book is for the parent who wants to show up for their career, their kids and their community, but isn't sure how to juggle it all.

This book is for those of us who want to claim their health again through simple changes that have a big impact.

If that's you, welcome.

Once you become clear and determined that time will not be the limiting factor in your health transformation; once you see that you can have reasons or results, but not both; once you choose conviction over convenience; once you look for the opportunity, not the obstacle; once you stop letting "perfect" be the enemy of "done"…

The world is going to get out of your way.

One tiny habit at a time.

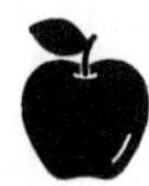

BOTTOM LINE:

- There is always an opportunity to enhance our wellbeing if one looks, plans, manages, and requests. Time and many obligations are malleable or negotiable.

- Many healthy habits can be executed in a matter of minutes, not hours. Seek the low-hanging fruit first.

- Start small. Start now.

- If you have trouble starting to exercise, visit **www.eattheapplebook.com** for a free workout guide.

Eat the apple

> **A seed hidden in the heart of an apple is an orchard invisible.**
>
> - Welsh Proverb

"Allyson? Is that you?"

"Derek?"

"Yes! Oh my gosh you look amazing!"

"Thank you, you too!"

Allyson was a former coworker from a restaurant job I'd had a lifetime prior. We ran into each other by chance at the same casino.

She was visibly trimmer, more vibrant... healthier.

After initial niceties about our current work and families, the topic turned back to her transformation.

"Most people don't look better as they age—you do! How does a single mom keep herself together so well?"

"You know me. Back in the day it was all booze, smoking, and hangover food."

"I happen to recall a similar lifestyle," I said with a smile.

If you're one of the current 17 million U.S. hospitality workers, you know this to be true.

"Yup! Call it maternal instincts, but after I got pregnant I knew I had to do better for my baby. I quit the booze and cigarettes. Cleaned up my diet as best I knew how at the time.

During Covid, I left the restaurant industry to focus on turning my side hustle into a full-time business. That gave me the space and time to focus further on my lifestyle decisions.

Once I wasn't surrounded by readily available food I really saw how much I left my nutritional choices to chance. Before, during my shift I'd have a few french fries here... a pita with spinach and artichoke dip there... There wasn't much rhyme or reason to my food selection at work. Whatever was there during work, I ate.

When I got responsible for all of my food decisions, I eventually hired a nutrition coach."

"Indeed! We can be helpful from time to time."

"I see that now!" Allyson quipped. "She helped me see that I could fill the gaps with some easily implementable changes."

"Like what?"

"Well, for example, I loved a croissant, egg, and cheese sandwich for breakfast. Tasty, but a lot of empty calories. Now I do a serving of blueberries and yogurt every morning. I can really feel the difference in how it makes my body feel for the rest of the day."

"That's amazing! The difference is clear... and you know, I felt the same thing once I switched from a junky granola bar to an apple for my midday snack. Fruit is a total upgrade over processed carbs."

"Totally. Don't get me wrong, I still enjoy the occasional baked goody—but I've found myself craving fruits and vegetables on the whole much more. It's even rubbed off on my daughter—she knows how to fuel herself with the good stuff before softball tournaments. Miles ahead of me at her age!"

"Amazing. Sometimes all it takes is one positive change to alter a legacy of health!"

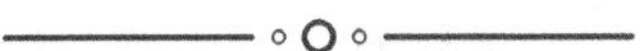

Fruit is the original sweet treat. When Adam said, "Don't bite the apple, Eve!" he wasn't saying so because apples weren't healthy.

To me, apples in particular may be the perfect food.

They've got fiber, vitamins and minerals, are high in water content, and have a slow blood sugar release. They travel well and keep for days without refrigeration.

Many people don't know apple flesh is high in quercetin (great for those sensitive to histamines or who have allergies), and the apple skins are high in pectin, which helps repair gut lining and offers other prebiotic fibers which feed beneficial gut bacteria.

Beyond those accolades, apples are an awesome marker for testing if I'm actually hungry (or just feeling snacky). They're tasty, but not so much that I overeat (though there are worse things to indulge in!). They're filling enough to satisfy for an hour or more without any guilt and stave off cravings for lesser foods.

Apples are my go-to foods before a workout.

On my best days I eat my apple. Doing so shows I was intentional enough to make healthy eating a priority. There are days I don't, and those days I usually end up wolfing down two bowls of sugary cereal instead.

Of course, you don't have to make apples the barometer of nutrition. Allyson chooses berries, an orange, or carrot sticks and hummus. One of my buddies eats an avocado per day... (Keto people, I tell ya!). These foods are all viable options.

Whatever you choose, make one serving of produce you love (or like well enough to eat most days) the staple of your snacking, and let that one choice be a nutritional baseline to achieve.

Most people only have 2-6 opportunities to eat per day. Making one food your litmus test of daily success (or at least partial success) is one of the easiest ways to develop a healthy routine.

BOTTOM LINE:

- Apples are awesome—the near-perfect snack.

- Choose your "apple" and make it a cornerstone of daily nutritional intake.

- Ask yourself, "Did I eat my apple today?" as a guidepost on your way to a healthier day.

Take the stairs

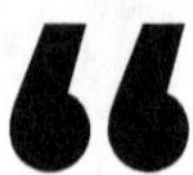

There are no traffic jams along the extra mile.

- Zig Ziglar

Fred was admittedly stuck... literally.

He liked to exercise with a trainer, but outside of that did very little.

"I literally do nothing without a trainer... I just don't think about exercising or moving about in my daily life."

A busy but sedentary job and no active hobbies had him peaking just a few pounds shy of the "300" club.

He was also stuck figuratively. After 30 years of marriage, he and his wife moved forward with a divorce. Through that stressful experience, he found a new lease on life and the desire to lose weight. (Funny how breakups can lead to inspired action.)

What began as walks around the neighborhood to get out of the house (they were still cohabiting until assets were divided) led to a relentless pursuit of getting more movement into each day. He gave up the golf cart and started walking the course. He finally found the stairwell in his office building ("I didn't know where it was for eight years!" he would say), and walked the stairs instead of using the elevator.

Needless to say, he dropped nearly 50 pounds and had to make space for a brand new wardrobe!

Funnily, he never did more "exercise" than before beyond the 2-3 sessions with his trainer. He was still a busy executive with all of the same responsibilities.

Fred simply chose to find the moments to move that were already available. He simply acted upon them. And that behavior change yielded compound interest far beyond an extra day per week in the gym.

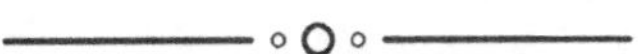

Extra movement throughout the day adds up fast.

Coined "N.E.A.T.," Non-Exercise Activity Thermogenesis is the secret weapon of the busy parent or professional. Why? Because physical activity—including both formal exercise and N.E.A.T.—accounts for 15-30% of total daily energy expenditure. For most people, formal exercise contributes negligibly to this number, while N.E.A.T. can account for most of their daily activity-related calorie burn.[1]

How? There's simply much more time in the day to move with intention.

If we sleep 8 hours, we're left with the other 16 to move, garden, pick up, put down, go the long way, etc.

Guess which one is more sustainable?

The longest-lived people on earth don't do CrossFit six times per week. They walk. A lot.

While strength training, increased cardiovascular output, and maximum exertion have their places, long-form gentle movement is the foundation to any exercise plan. There are also unique benefits to "non-exercise activity":

It's low intensity.

It's low injury-risk.

It feels good physically and mentally.

It can be done socially, promoting healthful connection with people above or below your abilities.

Consider this: walking will almost undoubtedly be your final access to exercise—with you until your dying days. Do it today so you can still do it at 100!

Walking and regular low intensity activity are two of the common practices among the longest-lived people across the world.

Use the pedometer on your phone (they all have them now) or buy a wearable tracker and track your steps. What may start out as taking just a few thousand (the average Westerner only takes around 3,500), will quickly increase to double or triple that with the simple practice of being aware of the metric and where you stand in relation to a step goal on a daily basis.

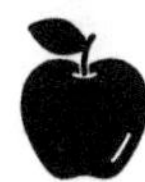

BOTTOM LINE:

- Weave movement throughout your day by making little choices to do so:

    - Park far away from the entrance.

    - Take the stairs to your office.

    - Walk to pick the kids up from school a few times per week.

    - Take a walking meeting instead of sitting in the office.

    - Do squats at your desk.

- Track your steps so you're aware of progress.

- Watch the pounds fall off.

Rethink your drink—minimize sugary beverages

I believe water is the only drink for a wise man.

- Henry David Thoreau

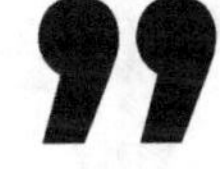

I was hired to do a corporate wellness event along with a few other practitioners of different skills.

While setting up next to a rep from a team-building company—a few hours before the event was to begin—we started making small talk. The conversation turned to health and fitness.

"You guys sure do look the brand—good on ya! I used to be pretty fit myself—gymnastics and acrobatics actually. Can't find the time to lose this spare tire anymore, though," he said as he grabbed his tummy pooch with both hands and shook it.

"Ahhh... I don't buy that, man. You just need to bring a few of those healthy habits back into existence again—you'll be fit as a fiddle in no time."

"Maybe. Even if I did start exercising again, it's just so expensive to eat healthy these days..."

Just a few minutes later, Max took a glass bottle out of his bag and drank some of its contents. It was a milky coffee drink from a leading chain. I got close enough to read the label.

"Frappuccino coffee drink... let's see what we're working with here..."

I quickly grabbed my phone to look up the nutrition contents.

9.5 ounces... 200 calories... 32 grams of sugar! That's 60% of the recommended daily value in one drink!

"Yeesh," I thought. "Max might not need to start any new habits, just stop a couple of old ones like this and he'll be back to fighting weight in no time."

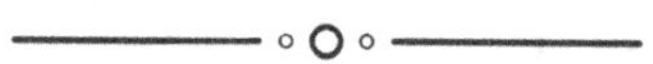

Sugar sweetened beverages are the leading source of added sugar in the American diet.

High-sugar beverages work against our waistline in a few ways:

Without fiber, protein, or really anything for our stomach to break down, sugary beverages create a near-instantaneous blood sugar spike upon entering the small intestine and liver, resulting in fat storage—even if we are moving vigorously while consuming.

Since they do nothing to satisfy our hunger (and even promote more hunger), we almost assuredly eat more calories throughout the day on top of the high calorie beverage.

Many brands contain other harmful ingredients such as food dyes, preservatives, or even other types of sugar our body has a harder time processing (such as high fructose corn syrup, which the liver stores as body fat when consumed in such high doses).

There are a host of other inflammatory issues related to sugary beverage consumption as well—diabetes, heart disease, tooth decay, among others.

Diet sodas and other drinks sweetened with sugar substitutes will still raise your blood sugar, lead to weight gain, and cause a host of other issues due to their synthetic nature.

There are a lot of arguments against consumption of sugary beverages, and I would be remiss not to say that just drinking water can be a bit... boring for some. Here are a few replacements that can flavor up your water without the consequences of sugary drinks:

Half of a sugar/artificial sweetener electrolyte packet serving — companies have come out with some tasty flavors as of late. They're also full of minerals and B vitamins (I like Trace Minerals, Prime, and Liquid IV).

Add a scoop of fruit & veggie powder — count it as an extra serving of daily produce if you're tracking!

Homemade iced teas — tons of health benefits here, especially squeezed with a lemon wedge for extra potassium. Prepare a large batch and store in the fridge to consume over a few days.

Carbonated waters/waters with gas — tasty effervescence! So many to choose from...

With so many quality sugar-free alternatives to choose from nowadays, this is an easy switch with a big upside.

BOTTOM LINE:

- Outside of eating out in restaurants less, cutting sugary drinks is the fastest way to drop a dress/pant size.

- "Diet" beverages with synthetic sweeteners can be even worse for your health and waistline.

- Making the switch away from sweetened drinks adds up to results fast; exchanging one can of soda for a zero sugar, healthier alternative equates to saving around 40 grams of sugar per day, 280 grams per week, 1,200 grams per month, and 14,400 grams per year!

Environment is everything

> # Our bodies are our gardens - our wills are our gardeners.
>
> – William Shakespeare

"That's a wrap—great job everyone!"

I had been hired by a company to conduct a team building event in which participants were separated into groups and assigned to do 10 silly events of varying ridiculousness in order to score points for their squad. In one such event, the employees had to get a cookie from their foreheads to their mouths without using their hands in 60 seconds. Good fun.

After the event was over, I was left with four extra packages of cookies.

Never one to waste food (if you can classify cookies as "food"), I was reluctant to throw these perfectly fresh, unused snacks away.

"You can save them and give them to unhoused people that you see in Los Angeles," my wife, who had helped me facilitate the event, said.

While cookies are far from the healthiest option to give to anyone, I figured perhaps better than hunger. And because I hate wasting food, it seemed like a fine idea at the time.

With that in mind, I faithfully put the cookies in a couple of paper bags in the front seat of my car, feeling good about the pure intentions to not only prevent food waste but also spread a little love in the world.

Fast-forward to the next week. I'm stuck in traffic on the way home. Not an unhoused person in sight.

What do my eyes see but a shiny blue package of chocolate chip cookies...

They were calling to me like a siren to the rocks.

Much as I tried to resist temptation, look away and focus on the road, the combination of being bored and a little anxious in traffic had me break down, tear open a package, and take one.

It was gone in seconds, as sweet treats often are.

Pandora's box had been opened and I was off to the races.

One turned into five.

In the snack attack I had consumed 325 empty calories in two minutes or less. It was swift and mindless indulgence.

A few minutes pass, traffic clears up, and shame for the junk food breakdown sets in.

"How could I, a health coach, not be able to take control of myself in the presence of temptation when it is an arm's reach away?! Tomorrow, I will give those cookies away to the first unhoused person I see and rid myself of them. Tomorrow I will be better."

The next day I'm driving and again get caught in traffic—lo and behold a particularly long bout of it. Couple that with the aftermath of a couple of stressful meetings, and I had found myself staring at the packages of cookies yet again. I had already eaten my pre-made lunch and snacks. I was left anxious and hungry.

They called to me with yet another test of my willpower.

I lost again.

Thirty minutes from home I broke down and ate. By the third cookie I had become more aware of my actions, but the damage was already done.

What's worse is that this occurred during my writing of this chapter!

That's right—I was in the middle of writing a health book with one of the most important chapters being about controlling one's environment for long-term health, fitness and aesthetics when this breakdown occurred.

The fact that I had consumed eight cookies in a matter of seconds spoke volumes about the importance of managing the environment for health, and my vulnerability when that environment is compromised.

I went for a shame run after the second binge and realized this is the perfect example to share the importance of maintaining the environment that supports one's goals... or to prepare to struggle and fail.

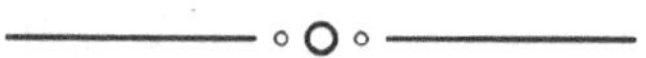

Epigeneticist and author Bruce Lipton said, "Just like a single cell, the character of our lives is determined not by our genes but by our responses to the environmental signals that propel life."[2]

Case in point: research conducted at Saint Bonaventure University found that when participants were offered both apple slices and buttered popcorn, they consumed significantly more of whichever food was placed within arm's reach—even when they reported preferring the taste of the food that was farther away.[3]

Think about what this means for your daily life. That buttered popcorn on your desk? You're not eating it because you're hungry or because you even want it that badly. You're eating it because it's there. Within arm's reach. Convenient.

The same principle works in reverse, though. Put the apple slices next to your workspace and move the popcorn to the cabinet across the room? Suddenly you're reaching for the apple without even thinking about it.

These aren't huge, dramatic changes. But they add up. An extra 100 calories of candy per day—roughly what you'd consume from mindless desk snacks—becomes an extra pound every month. That's 12 pounds by the end of the year, or about one dress or pant size.

All from proximity.

If faced with temptation, we simply cannot overcome our surroundings long-term (or even short-term in my case). Healthy or unhealthy, we'll almost certainly rise and fall with our surroundings and our tribe.

The Hawthorne effect describes how people modify their behavior when they're being watched. Add social pressure—our desire to look good and belong—and we're even more likely to act differently around others.

I'll use my wife as an example. She is dedicated to portion control. I've never seen her overeat. She literally nibbles on pumpkin seeds out of a ramekin for a snack.

So, you can see with a life partner who adheres to that level of rigor, my habit of eating until uncomfortably full is mitigated simply by being in her presence (I wish she had been in the car with me during my solo cookie binges!).

It continues to bring home the point that maintaining an environment (and the people in it) that supports our health goals is paramount—a foundational starting point to any health transformation.

BOTTOM LINE:

- Before beginning a new wellness venture, have a look in your pantry and fridge—ensure the food is 90% nutrient rich, calorically low, and easy to access/consume.

- Take inventory of the food scene at work. Are there healthy snack and meal options? If not, it may be time to bring your own.

- Notice if your life allows for opportunities to move. If you're confined to a desk, consider how to overcome limited mobility with planned movement breaks throughout the day.

- Make being healthy even easier by enrolling your partner, friends, and family into the same vision (or to at least support you in yours!).

Thank your God immediately upon waking

> In the morning, Lord, you hear my voice; in the morning I lay my requests before you and wait expectantly.
>
> - Psalm 5:3

In 2015 I hit a rough patch. My girlfriend and I broke up; I was partying too much, not learning anything new, and living in a miserable, roach-infested apartment off of Vermont Avenue. I was walking in a cloud of malaise.

Days rolled into weeks and I continued to feel stuck—doing and thinking the same patterns over and over again.

After a particularly rollicking weekend to drown my blues away, I received a lightning bolt from the Heavens above:

"You. You are choosing this life, and not choosing to see the joy and abundance I provide you. Choose gratitude, love of self, and love of others every morning and all will change."

At that moment I closed my eyes, put one hand on my heart, the other in the sky toward God, smiled and thanked them. I thanked them for my health, the work I had to pay my bills, for good friends and family, for the sun and moon and oxygen to breathe and food to eat and to live in a beautiful city. In that beaming moment I got that everything I need is already laid before me—I just need to look and acknowledge it.

Years later, still every morning when I wake up, before my feet touch the ground, without fail, I will put one hand on my heart, the other to the sky toward God, smile and thank them for the life bestowed upon me with a short prayer:

"Heavenly father, earth mother, thank you for this day. Thank you for abundance, prosperity, and joy. Thank you for family, thank you for friends. Thank you for the opportunity to show up big for my dreams today. Thank you for everything you provide and continue to provide. Let's make today magical, let's make today fun. In your name I pray, I pray, I pray, amen."

Some mornings I add other things I'm grateful for, but typically just that micro prayer. And it's always steered me on a course of happiness, patience, and connection to others and to God for the day.

Challenges still arise throughout my days but every morning I choose to begin with peace. And that has made all the difference.

———————— ∘ O ∘ ————————

People always ask me, "How are you ALWAYS in a good mood? You simply can't fake it for this long!"

While it's true I've had a happy disposition from childhood, even the innately content still experience throes of sadness, depression, anxiety, loathing or any other bitter flavor life feeds us at some point.

Any one or combination of those emotions can color a day, week, a month, or even a lifetime, of someone who is left unconscious to their impact. We embody our thoughts. Over time, negative emotions can pull us away from God source.

We need a daily anchor to ground us in our body and connect to the divine so we can move through the day with the right mindset.

Enter a gratitude practice very (very) first thing in the morning.

Spiritual channeler Esther Hicks says the brief space between unconscious (sleep/meditation) and consciousness (waking) holds the greatest opportunity to change our mood and outlook going forward—the chance to "uplevel" our vibration and leave behind any residue of the past that weighs us down.

And in my experience, they're right.

The fleeting moments between sleep and wakefulness bring us the greatest chance to choose how we'll think and behave for the day, no matter what lies ahead.

Consider waking as the blank slate to start fresh and a morning prayer to put God and positive expectations in your heart.

See for yourself and come up with your own morning prayer; check out the next page to view a Mad-Libs style starter script, handy for those who haven't prayed much before.

Morning Prayer

Dear (*your noun for God*),

....

Thank you for today.
Thank you for this (*noun*)

....

....

....

Thank you for my (*noun of something you already have*)

....

....

....

Thank for being able to (*verb for something you enjoy*)

....

....

....

Please guide me toward (*enter what you'd like to focus attention
on for the day, week, month, year, life.*)

....

....

....

And how I may be in service to (*a group that matters to you.*)

....

....

....

Thank you for the power to overcome (current challenge);

....

....

....

and (anything else to be grateful for?)

....

....

....

And for the gift my life is.
Let's make today (adjective).

....

....

....

Let's make today (adjective).

....

....

....

In your name I pray, **Amen** (or other spiritual completion noun).

....

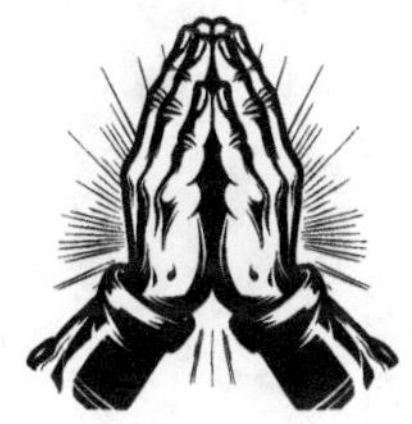

Make it your own, of course. And speak it in such a way that you embody the words you choose—it will help you live the message throughout the day. Smiling wholeheartedly as you pray truly helps. Even if you have to fake it at first, it will still elevate feel-good serotonin levels.

Once you see the practice bear fruit in subsequent waking hours, you'll have yet another reason to give thanks next time you begin a new day.

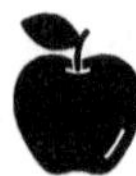

BOTTOM LINE:

- The moment just after we wake up is the perfect moment to influence our mood for the day.

- Saying a prayer and giving gratitude is a choice we can all make. No matter what breakdown is occurring in our lives when we are here on this planet, it is a privilege to live the life of comfort that we do.

- Smiling, hand on heart while praying, brings the spoken word to life. Take thirty seconds to say it with conviction every morning.

Be Fully Self-Expressed

> # If you can walk you can dance, if you can talk you can sing.
>
> - Zimbabwean proverb

"I just can't sing, and that's that," my wife said on a holiday evening with family after the kids went to sleep.

"Bull. What makes you say that?" I retorted.

"I tried once when I was a kid. My dad and sister said it was terrible."

"So... your dad and sister, neither of which are professional singers nor vocal coaches, gave their amateur opinion, and you took it to heart as an adolescent... and haven't sung since?"

"Yep."

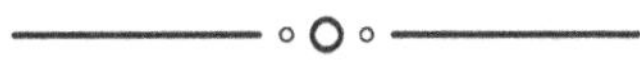

This story has been an annoyance of mine for the last ten years.

It's a shining example of limiting oneself (or accepting limitations others put upon us), cutting off any possibility of improving the skill set we possess, or sidelining ourselves from the simple pleasure in the act of moving and making noise.

Anthropologist Angeles Arrien says that African shamans may ask patients questions like, "When in your life did you stop singing?" and "When in your life did you stop dancing?" when trying to figure out a patient's diagnosis.

My aunt has a print of a Zimbabwean proverb at her house. It reads: "If you can walk you can dance, if you can talk, you can sing."

It always struck me as a beautiful way to say, "Jump in, no matter what it sounds or looks like—you and others will be glad you did."

Singing and dancing are pure human expressions of joy. They make you an active participant in life. No wallflowers here. Peer-reviewed research has demonstrated dancing's benefits for hearts, lungs, and waistlines (c'mon, Zumba!). Singing supports heart and lung health too, though more gently.[4] Above and beyond that, singing and dancing are good for mental health—good for the soul.

Being generous and playful in a given moment goes far beyond us—it gives permission for others to do the same, spreading happiness far and wide.

No one says you have to strive to be great, or even good at either. I've got two decent dance moves I do on repeat and never had a choral solo in high school music class. Doing both rudimentarily still brings me happiness and I do them often.

If you're stunted in any form of creative self expression, ask: "Where does that blockage come from?"

And once you've pegged that down to a memory or preconceived belief, ask: "Is it true?"

Whether it is or it isn't is inconsequential—being in approval of yourself in the creative act matters most! Break through any fear and be delighted in the newfound self-expression when you begin.

BOTTOM LINE:

- Life is too short to let teasing or self-imposed limitations stop us from singing, dancing, and being fully self-expressed.

- Sometimes a little bit of self-expression and play can do more for our health than anything else.

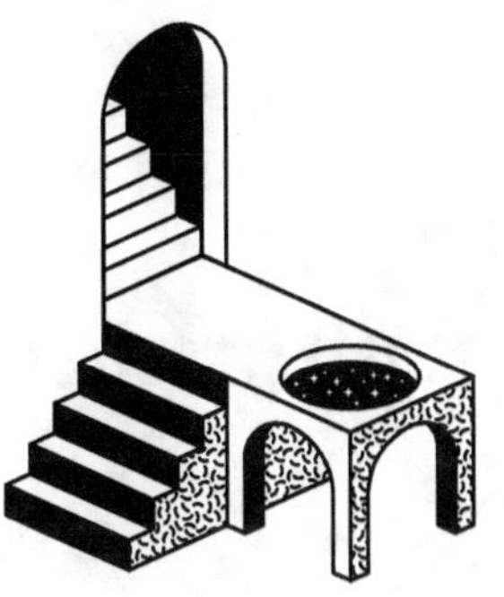

SECOND FLIGHT

Move after eating

42 | EAT THE APPLE, TAKE THE STAIRS

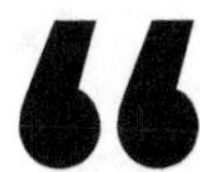

> # If you take 100 steps after each meal, you'll live to 99.
>
> – Chinese folk wisdom

After a long day of testing, the doctor called with news:

"Your blood work has come back, Kristen—unfortunately you've failed the second glucose test, which means we're diagnosing you with gestational diabetes."**

Kristen is a dear friend and, at that time, a mother expecting her first child.

"Okay, so what do we do about that?" Kristen replied nervously.

"Well, first we'll need to set you up with blood glucose monitors—both finger sticks and a continuous glucometer to make sure you and the baby stay within safe ranges and keep this pregnancy without complications." The doctor went on…

"I don't want to put you on medication if possible, so Julie will be going over the lifestyle changes we recommend that can keep the blood sugar in check," he said, referring to the nurse also on the call.

"Yes, much we can do," Julie said, now leading the conversation. "We'll want you to tightly monitor your diet: carbohydrates, especially grains—less is better in most instances. Fats are slower burning energy, so olive oils, avocado, and whole fat yogurt are good options. Stay away from the fried oils, however. High protein and vegetables should be the cornerstone of your diet for now. We'll need you to keep a comprehensive food journal, as well as record the times you're eating and the post-meal blood sugar data you get."

"Oh wow… and okay, yes… anything else?" Kristen asked.

"Yes. Outside of nutrition and keeping stress low, the most important practice to regulate blood sugar spikes after meals is to walk."

"Just… walk?"

"Yes, studies show that five to ten minutes of walking can lower post-meal blood sugar," said nurse Julie. "It doesn't have to be only walking, either. Gentle stretching, cleaning up the house, a few gentle body weight exercises… just don't sit for 5-10 minutes immediately after eating."

Kristen felt like this was something she could do, and was now experiencing a little hope after receiving some potentially concerning news.

With a focus on increased protein and vegetable intake, fewer carbohydrates and moving after every meal, Kristen was able to better manage her gestational diabetes and deliver a beautiful son.

"I can't believe how much moving after meals supported my blood sugar and well-being while pregnant," she told me. "Doing it conceptually made sense, but I just never thought to make it a practice—until I had to. To this day I still prioritize walking after meals because of the experience!"

**Gestational diabetes is a form of glucose intolerance that occurs during pregnancy and typically resolves after pregnancy.

Postprandial movement is not a new phenomenon. Ancient Ayurvedic medicine text called for the practice of "shatapavali" or "walking 100 steps" after every meal to aid one to live to 100 years old.

Walking is so effective at managing blood sugar that a meta-analysis found 2-5 minutes was enough to "smooth" glucose spikes and reduce the risk of developing type 2 diabetes.[1]

Walking also strengthens digestion by stimulating contractions of the digestive tract and improving blood flow to the area.

If weather or family duties won't let you outside for a brief period, simply walk about the house, clean, do dishes, play with the kids or pets... all can be excellent ways to get some post-meal non-exercise activity. Whatever you do, stay off the couch for a few extra minutes and move!

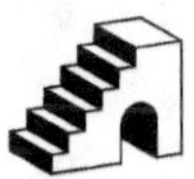

BOTTOM LINE:

- A few minutes of movement after meals can have a statistically significant impact on reducing blood sugar spikes.

- If walking after eating can help diabetics in such a short amount of time, it can surely help busy moms, dads and professionals just like you stay a little healthier, too.

Make yourself a morning smoothie

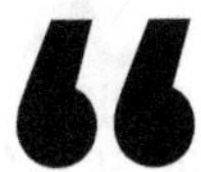

Smoothies - the best way to trick your kids into eating their vegetables.

- Derek Opperman

The American breakfast started as a marketing ploy by pork companies to sell more products. It has no beneficial effects for our bodies.

"If you really want to level up your and your clients' morning routines, you've got to consider a smoothie to break your fast," my first integrative health teacher would preach. "Our body isn't designed for that kind of food first thing in the morning. We need to hydrate and slowly wake up the digestive tract, not bombard it with pork or sugar."

This was news to me. I had been a bacon and eggs guy since I started cooking for myself.

Processed breakfast meat, usually pork sausage, 4-6 eggs and 2-3 pieces of toast with lots of butter... sometimes all of it drizzled with cheese. What's not to love? How about:

- The daily recommended amount of sodium in just one meal

- Highly processed, oxidized, carcinogenic animal flesh

- A hard-to-process first meal of the day for the digestive tract

- Three of the top food sensitivities in one meal (eggs, dairy, gluten/ wheat).

Quite a way to start the day!

All of these ingredients are delicious and even beneficial if of good quality and consumed at the right time. A big American breakfast is still one of my weekend joys.

It's just not necessarily the healthiest option to regularly employ first thing in the morning.

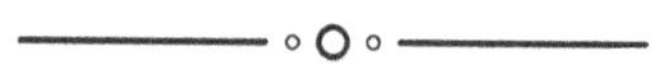

When done cleanly and correctly, smoothies are:

- Hydrating

- High in fruit, vegetable and fiber count

- High in protein, vitamins and minerals

- Healthy fats

- Easy to digest as a first meal

Let's have a quick look at each one of these benefits:

Hydrating: When we wake up in the morning we're dehydrated—our bodies use up to a liter of water when we sleep for respiration, perspiration, detoxification, and digestion. Depending on what study you look at, a significant portion of adults (skewing older) are chronically dehydrated.

Drinking enough fluids ensures we remain the roughly 60% water we're supposed to be composed of. Your brain? 80% water. Kidneys? 80%. Even your heart and lungs are about 75% water.[2]

While I extol the virtues of a glass of water first thing in the morning, a smoothie reinforces the hydration habit and offers a myriad of other benefits when our body is ready to refuel.

High fruit and vegetable count: Ninety percent of people don't get the recommended five or more fruits and vegetables per day... ninety percent! Eighty-eight percent fall short on fruit. The bar isn't even high—we're talking 2-3 cups of vegetables and 1.5-2 cups of fruit per day.[3]

To me, fruits and vegetables should truly be the base of our food pyramid (what we consume the most). No other food group can match their antioxidant count, fiber, vitamin and mineral levels and more. They're generally high in nutrients and low in caloric density (and trust me, it's not the sweet fruits that are driving our obesity epidemic). A properly made smoothie will check off two or more of those five servings and bring your body the quality, sustained energy it deserves.

High-protein, nutrient-dense meal replacement powders: Meal replacement powders have come a long way since I started choking them down in the late 90's. Now we've got a world of delicious, quality options to suit our tastes and preferences.

Quick aside: due to destructive farming practices over the last 60 years, the quality of our soil has plummeted, and in turn so has the nutrient content of our food.[4] Because of this we're getting far less of the necessary vitamins and minerals, even if we have the best dietary intentions. Enter meal replacement powder—formulated supplements that hold a spectrum of the nutrients our standard American diet is missing.

Look for one that contains a high amount of vitamins, minerals and protein (whey, hemp, pea, rice or a blend can all be viable options, pending your dietary restrictions). Add a half cup of zero sugar, unsweetened yogurt per serving to further boost protein and satiety. You may want to skip this step if you have a weak digestive constitution; mixing dairy and fruit can be hard for some people if they don't pass it fast enough. As with anything, the quality of these products varies greatly. Do your due diligence and choose a brand which tests for heavy metals and has a Certificate of Analysis (CoA) to prove it.

Healthy fats: Quality fats are essential for brain health, heart health, cellular structure, vitamin absorption, inflammation management, and much more. Good fats can also be tough to find out in the world, so adding them to a daily smoothie ensures their consumption and your optimization. Flax seed powder, full-fat yogurt/kefir, avocado, or MCT oil are quality additions to a smoothie.

Easy to digest: Smoothie ingredients are blended, which makes them "pre-digested," and they're therefore easier for our bodies to process. This is more important than many people realize.

Our organs wake up in the morning, just like we do... sometimes they're a little slow to come to! Wolfing down a sausage, egg, and cheese sandwich while rushing off to work just isn't the best option (especially if you're a slow/late riser). For most people, digestive strength peaks between 11am and 2pm, but I typically don't recommend waiting that long to break a fast. Consuming something light and healthy in the morning is great to cut stress/cortisol and re-up depleted nutrients. And smoothies fit the bill for this perfectly.

Invest in a large capacity blender (we like Ninja), which will allow you to make up to 72 ounces of smoothie at once, saving time and making enough for three or four servings.

Here's my daily recipe (makes 3-4 servings):

- 24 ounces nut milk

- 24 ounces purified water

- 6 scoops EquiLife meal replacement powder

- 4 cups organic mixed frozen berries (Costco)

- 4 cups organic fresh baby spinach or kale (Costco)

- 1/4 cup MCT oil

- 1.5 cup unsweetened whole fat organic yogurt or 1 cup no sugar added Kefir (I don't blend the kefir, just add it after to keep probiotics alive).

Blend until smooth.

This mix gives me nearly every base nutrient I need to function in daily life, together with 25-30 grams of protein and quality fat for brain health. It's hydrating and delicious while still being low in sugar!

While you can certainly adjust for taste or goal, the practice only takes about ten minutes from start (ingredients out) to finish (ingredients away and blender cleaned), and if you do it in bulk you only need to do it every few days. Did I mention the total cost is only about half that of a Starbucks coffee and pastry?

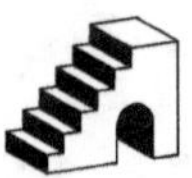

BOTTOM LINE:

- When done correctly, a morning smoothie checks off so many boxes:

  - Hydrating.

  - Vitamin, mineral, and protein rich.

  - Two servings of fruits and vegetables.

  - Inexpensive (when you make it yourself).

  - Time-saving (when done in bulk).

  - It's a can't-miss start to one's day.

- Need some smoothie inspiration? Visit **www.eattheapplebook.com** for a free downloadable smoothie recipe guide.

Hydrate and bathe with as pure water as possible

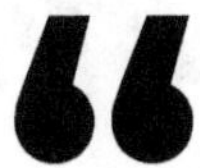

> # When the well is dry,
> # we know the value of water.
>
> - Benjamin Franklin

"Hmmmm, this water tastes weird."

I noticed something was "off" when I moved to Los Angeles and poured a glass of water from the Brita filter.

It was hard to explain, but the water had a texture and aftertaste unlike what I was used to from the mineral-rich, rural well water back in Connecticut. It certainly didn't feel hydrating.

The water still tasted funny even after changing the jug's filter.

Little did I know our well-intentioned Brita was ill-equipped to handle the myriad contaminants lurking in the Los Angeles water supply...

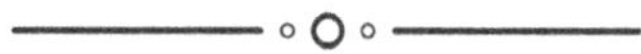

For humans having a firm-ish looking body, we sure are made of a high proportion of water.

Sixty to sixty-five percent of the skin is composed of water. 75-80% of the brain and muscles are composed of water. 80-85% of the lungs are composed of water. Heck, even our bones are 25-30% water, and they're among the hardest parts of bodies. Teeth? 8-10% water—and tooth enamel is the hardest substance we've got.[5]

From that perspective, it's easy to see the paramount importance of having water available to replenish our entire body. But just as necessary, we must have pure water available.

So, I was shocked when I discovered that my home's tap water had cancer-causing Arsenic at 10 times the legal limit, and 275x higher levels than the Environmental Working Group's water safety standards!

Perhaps even more concerning was that there were many other contaminants found in my home's water that weren't even given a safe legal limit by the Environmental Protection Agency (EPA), meaning governing bodies aren't entirely sure how toxic certain substances found in our water are to us.

Most alarming of all, these contaminant levels aren't considered dangerous—in fact, they're completely acceptable American standards!

This speaks to the fact America hasn't updated its clean water standards in over 20 years and doesn't have the federal oversight to enforce necessary regulations even when they do.

Legal doesn't equal safe. Just ask Flint, Michigan and Jackson, Mississippi, who were drinking lead and arsenic-infused water for years, distributed freely by local municipalities until infrastructure tragedies exposed their toxicity.

Dirty tap water coming out of our faucets is more common than most realize. It's crucial to ensure you're consuming as few contaminants as possible.

And before you simply reach for the bottled water, studies show 93% of brands contain plastic particles. One bottle? Over 10,000 pieces per liter.[6]

Your best bet is to secure a high-quality filter or filtration system (and no, the filter in your fridge probably won't cut it).

Here are a few I like for quality and cost at the time of writing:

For countertop filters, I like Cyclone products—good for individuals. I can taste the difference.

For under sink installed filters, I like AquaTru's reverse osmosis system—good for families, though this one does require a plumber.

For external units (no plumbing required), I like Primo units. You can often find Primo water filling stations close to your local grocer or drug store.

For shower and bath filtration, I like Crystal Quest products—certified and made in the USA.

How do I know which filter to choose?

Your needs will differ depending on where you live, so it's best to discover what your needs are first before purchasing a filter.

Go to https://www.ewg.org/tapwater/system, type in your zip code and discover which contaminants are in your local municipal water supply.

From there you can ascertain which type of filter you need by viewing EWG's filter recommendations.

When purchasing, look for the National Sanitation Foundation (NSF) certified label, which ensures the filter meets water treatment standards and the product passes certain performance requirements to earn the grade.

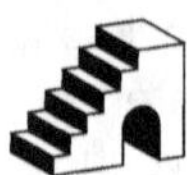

BOTTOM LINE:

- Humans are composed of approximately 60% water, with many organs composed of much higher amounts than that.

- We need to replenish water stores every day for optimal health.

- Our body literally becomes what we consume over months and years; thus, it only makes sense we should prioritize consuming the very best quality water possible.

- There are too many contaminants lurking in our tap water to be complacent on this one.

Got a few minutes? Get outside, shoes off

> **My own prescription for health is less paperwork and more running barefoot through the grass.**
>
> - Terri Guillemets

Regan is a family friend with a wild story.

She grew up with divorced parents. Alcoholism in the home. Chronic stress from living through generational dysfunction. And she overcame those odds in her youth to become a high-level athlete (she swam the English Channel... while pregnant!) and obtain her Master of Fine Arts. She also held a steady job and raised three healthy, well-adjusted children of her own. It was important to look good, be perceived as successful, have it all together in spite of her past. But through all the perceived success, she had a critical sense of self, and never felt like she fit in.

The burden of perfectionism has a price.

In 2018 Regan hit a wall.

Within a year, one brother died of a drug overdose. Then she lost another by suicide. She got divorced. To top it off, she was diagnosed with stage 3 breast cancer in one breast, then another. Her once sculpted physique and curated beauty were ravaged by harsh cancer drugs.

"At one point I had nothing left but a soul," she told me.

Any one of those experiences would be enough to bury a person in depression and angst.

While working her way through chemotherapy, Regan was called to the woods, to the grounding and healing vibration of nature. She made a vow with her favorite tree: "Please help heal me so I can help heal you."

From there, she made it a daily practice to be in nature. Sometimes the chemo wouldn't allow her to be outside in the sun for long, but, regardless, every day she allowed herself the time to be "bathed" by the sounds, smells, and sights of the forest.

"This newfound relationship with nature slowed my life down. It created the space to be present to the miracle of the natural world around me. It opened me to awe, beauty, and wonder. I came alive inside. I am certain my forest bathing practice helped me heal from cancer and get me through the trauma of the year gone by."

Fast forward seven years and Regan is cancer free. She has upheld her agreement with the forest and now leads nature walks with people who seek to anchor themselves within its rejuvenating vibrations and develop a different relationship to the great outdoors. She's even opened a school to teach inspired practitioners on how to do the same.

"We don't have to go away into a forest to have an experience like this," she says. "Nature is everywhere. It is the intentional appreciation of our natural world that centers our soul. It can be simply getting your feet in the grass, touching and observing a vegetable, taking a few deep breaths of the morning air. Slow down. Be present and open to the ever-present wonder around us."

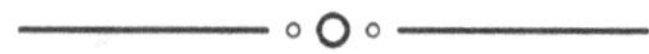

Humanity is going out far less than it used to. A study by the EPA found that people spend 87% of their time indoors, with another 6% of daily time spent in a car. That's 93% of our entire life![7]

With so much work to do at our desks and so many conveniences in our home (Netflix and chill is a lifestyle, man!), Western humanity has forgotten that there are so many easy, pleasurable and free health benefits to getting outside.

I'll start by reinforcing a few benefits of the great outdoors you may have already heard of (but it's always a good reminder!):

Sunshine: Full spectrum light rays from the sun support us by helping our body produce vitamin D, which improves bone density, immunity, and mood. Getting outside on a lunch break (or between 10am and 2pm, without sunscreen for most people) provides peak UVB rays crucial for vitamin D production. Start with 10 minutes of maximum skin exposure, and work your way up to 30 minutes, depending on personal skin tone and tolerance.[8]

Fresh(er) air: Due to paint/furniture outgassing, chemicals, and aerosol sprays used to "clean" our homes and workplaces, and generally more stagnant airflow, indoor air is regularly 2-5x more toxic than outdoor air—and can be up to 100x more toxic under certain conditions.[9]

Less screen interaction: While our phones are ever-present, TV's and desktops don't come with us outside, further reducing screen exposure and sparing our eyes from the strain blue light puts upon them for hours on end.

Yet there are still other wins the masses miss when it comes to benefits of the great outdoors:

Feet in grass/earth: Think about the last time you took your shoes off and put bare feet in the grass or sand. I'd bet it hasn't been often, and assert it hasn't been frequent enough for most readers. Skin-to-ground contact with the earth is reported to support improved sleep quality by way of higher heart rate variability (a good thing) and reduced inflammation, among other benefits.[10]

Resets circadian rhythm: Getting outside helps suppress melatonin in the morning (with or without direct sunshine), waking us up naturally. To that end, an evening stroll at dusk helps calm our nervous system, increasing melatonin and preparing us for sleep. That little walk after dinner also promotes digestion—another rest support.

Better posture: You've heard the popular saying, "Sitting is the new smoking." Getting outside tends to keep us upright and thus in better natural alignment without chronic strain on our neck, hips, and lower back. Other clinical benefits include reduced blood pressure and improved focus and cognition. Studies show working memory and attention consistently improve after nature exposure, even brief visits.[11]

And the beautiful thing is, you get all these benefits at once in a few short minutes!

Nowadays, there's almost nothing more satisfying and rejuvenating to me than coming home from work, taking off my shoes, and playing with my kids outside in the backyard. The habit checks off so many boxes, it's a hard one to reason missing out on. I encourage you to start a practice of getting outside (shoes off!) in whatever fashion your environment allows.

If you can get to a forest or park, great. If it's simply your backyard, great. If you're an urban dweller without much green, at the very least find the time to get sun on a lunch break. It makes a difference. Trust me (and Regan) on this one.

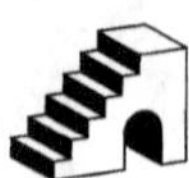

BOTTOM LINE:

- A healthy dose of sunshine, fresh(er) air, and movement check off so many boxes at once—a true healthy habit stack!

- Get maximum skin exposure when the season allows.

- Bonus points for getting your feet in grass or bare earth.

- 10-20 minutes per day is all you need.

Pomodoro technique— mastering alarm setting so you can have a better work/health balance

> **Almost everything will work again if you unplug it for a few minutes, including you.**
>
> - Anne Lamott

"Sometimes I would find myself sitting at my desk from breakfast through lunch... not getting up once beyond a bathroom break... just working for hours on end."

As an attorney practicing tort law, Michael had to read and actively interpret hundreds of pages of documents for a case, and often had multiple cases going on simultaneously. That's a lot of unchecked sitting time!

Not only that, it's also intense work with deadlines and big money at stake. Something he missed could cost his clients millions of dollars. That's a lot of stressed out sitting time!

"I would stomp around my office in a negative state for hours, just slogging through work and cursing everything—the deadlines with endless pages of discovery to read, my incompetent co-workers, my opposing counsel... With this attitude, I could see my mental health suffer and my quality of work suffer. I was taking shortcuts to survive until the end of the day. This being the nature of my work, I had to do something."

That's when Mike discovered the Pomodoro technique—a method of working 25 minutes and breaking for 5 minutes, repeated twice every hour, using alarms set throughout the day to remind oneself to get up and move.

"Setting and abiding by physical alarms to get up and move really made the difference. I need the reminder to stop and smell the roses—if I don't use them, I revert right back to working hours on end without getting up. Plus, I come back to my work refreshed and ready to perform. It's not always just walking. Sometimes I'll do a chore, stretch a little, get some sun. Whatever I do, I know I'm now consistently getting 7,000-9,000 steps—double what I'd otherwise get without setting movement reminders."

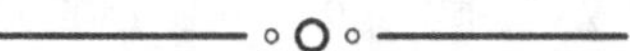

The sedentary work lifestyle is causing a bipedal epidemic.

With the advent of computers and digital work, 4 in 10 jobs are now defined as "sedentary," and the average American only takes around 3,000 to 4,000 steps per day (when it's said our ancestors walked closer to 10,000-18,000). It's clear why the lack of movement during waking hours is one of the main culprits as to why nearly 3 out of 4

Americans are overweight or obese.[12]

I see this all the time with my business professional clients: desk-bound from morning meetings through lunch (eaten at their desks, of course) straight into afternoon meetings and tasks. Suddenly it's 5pm. They've taken 2,200 steps. This isn't the exception. It's the norm.

We're moving far less than we should as locomotive human beings —Americans average only about one-third the daily steps of modern hunter-gatherers. Lack of movement impacts more than weight. Poor digestion, constricted circulation, improper posture, impacted mood and cognition, and low vitamin D levels are all consequences of insufficient daily movement (especially outside).[13]

We've got to get proactive if we are to overcome this cultural inertia.

Enter the Pomodoro technique—a time blocking structure composed of 25 minutes of dedicated, focused work, followed by a 5-10 minute break to leave the desk.

Pomodoro technique has supported clients to manage their physical and mental well-being—much more than the unconscious, sedentary American work routine they typically employ.

Of course, that 25:5 time structure isn't set in stone. One can stretch it to 45-50 minutes of work with a longer, 15 minute break to round out the hour if needed. Either way, aim to move 10-15 minutes within every hour of work.

It's simple: all you need to do is set up an automatic alarm on your phone every 25/45 minutes and get up and move when it goes off. If you've got a health tracker/wearable, you can automatically set these timers (and track those steps per day, too).

Consider the average person takes 90-120 steps per minute. If one takes 10 minutes to walk, that's an extra 900-1200 steps per hour. Multiply that by eight working hours, and that's an extra 7,200-9,600 steps per day. If this is implemented, the sedentary crisis is solved.

And I'd bet you'll be more productive too! The dedicated work:rest ratio supports my practicing clients and me to stay fresh and engaged for much longer than marathon bouts of work with no end in sight. We're left empowered, not fully beholden to endless tasks.

In fact, the great philosopher Aristotle believed he did his best thinking while walking. His peripatetic philosophy (meaning "given to walk about") had him and his students moving about the Lyceum discussing ethics and government.

Truthfully, it's hard to find a reason not to walk more. Sometimes we just need a few nudges to get going.

So the next time you feel overwhelmed with a cumbersome to-do list, try the Pomodoro technique. You'll go from saying, "I don't have time to move," to "How much time do I have to move?"

The answer and outcome may surprise and delight you!

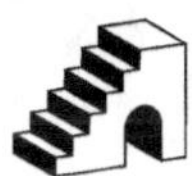

BOTTOM LINE:

- Setting alarms to move once or twice every hour of work will dramatically support maintaining healthy weight and body function without going to the gym every day.

- Peripatetic movement can even help us tackle challenging work problems.

- Have a dignified look at the time you have available in your day and schedule in your movement blocks (make them a different color for quick identification).

- The practice will give you freedom and flexibility. You'll be amazed how much gets done, and the satisfaction that comes along with it.

Celebrate, record, and remember your wins

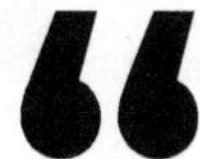

Victory is not won in miles, but in inches.

- Louis L'Amour

"Yeah man, the holidays make me more appreciative than ever, knowing how close I was to throwing my whole life away."

Shorty was a fellow graduate of a coaching program we had done together. We reconnected around Thanksgiving one year through an alumni networking event. I knew him, but didn't *know* him, ya dig? This was our first time talking about something not related to our program.

"What do you mean?" I asked, holding a napkin in one hand and a small plate of finger food in the other.

"Well, let's just say I had a hard home life. My parents only knew how to discipline me by whooping me. And that led me to believe I had to prove how tough I was, how much respect I got by taking a beating— and giving a beating right back."

I quickly saw our upbringings were miles apart.

"So I started to run the streets. I got involved with a gang. Fighting, drinking, selling, defending our turf. I was small, but made sure everyone knew I was not to be crossed."

By this point Shorty was already down memory lane, leaving me and this pleasant holiday party miles away.

"I literally fought my way to notoriety. I was the hardest dude in my corner of the city. I fought other gang members, but also friends and family. I eventually found myself with the money and respect I thought I always wanted, but no one wanted to be around me. They were terrified of me. Waking up alone from a drunken stupor one morning, I remember how lonely that felt.But I wasn't about to slow down. Until I did. I caught my first sentence at 14."

"Whaaatttt?" I said in disbelief.

I couldn't believe it. Little as I personally knew Shorty, he always emanated love to me. It was hard to accept he had that side in him.

"For real. I did two and a half years with leniency for a first-time offense. But I didn't learn a damn thing. I was in and out of prison for a decade."

Shorty went on.

"I hit rock bottom when I got blacked out drunk and woke up in a jail cell with no idea how I got there. At that point I had two young sons. I realized this isn't me anymore. I was throwing away my potential and my life. It was at that moment that I just prayed to God to keep me safe and get me home to my boys.

The judge was merciful and only gave me two and a half years. But he looked me in the eye and said this is my last chance—if he saw me again, it was going to be along with a sentence that had me locked up for much, much longer."

My mouth was agape.

"So I did my time," Shorty went on.

"When I got out I knew I had to make good on my promise to God, the judge, and myself. I joined AA, did therapy, and worked hard on healing relationships. Trust me, it wasn't easy—all that selfishness, all the pain I had caused required so much forgiveness."

"Wow. Yeah, I can see how much it must've taken to clean up your life to that extent. How were you able to stay on the straight and narrow for all these years?" I asked.

"There were a lot of factors, man. But one of the many tools I learned in Alcoholics Anonymous was that our past is the best asset if it's utilized properly. So, at night I began to revisit the conversations I had that day through a journaling practice. I reflected on moments when my anger would get the best of me, and I would celebrate the victories when I let love and patience lead the way."

"So you just... journal?"

"Yeah, it's wild for me, a kid from the 'hood, to say that. But once I stopped resisting my soul's call to record my feelings, I've found the daily writing and gratitude practice to be so healing. I get to acknowledge my victories and keep the amends I need to make alive and in existence. It's part of the spiritual workout I do daily. And I am clear it's made me a better boss, father, and person."

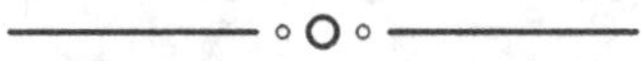

Much as I've tried, keeping a gratitude journal like Shorty just hasn't stuck for me.

While the habit hasn't become routine, I do love looking back on past entries. It's such a joy to be teleported back to moments in time and glimpse what I was thinking, doing, and being—however many years ago.

But alas, finding a time to keep a gratitude journal continues to elude me.

Enter the Jar of Awesome—a simple substitute to regular gratitude journaling if you crave something similar like I did.

Popularized by best-selling author Tim Ferriss, a Jar of Awesome "is a well-being practice where you write down memories representing positive experiences, accomplishments, and revisit them when needed, fostering a sense of gratitude and reminding you of your awesomeness."

All you need is a jar, some post-its, and a pen.

Whenever something positive happens worth remembering, simply jot it down on a post-it and drop in the jar. I add the date as a reference as well.

The practice is powerful for big, peak life events (having a successful IVF cycle with a surrogate), and also smaller ones that we might otherwise not remember (setting a personal exercise record, finally having a hard conversation you were avoiding, receiving a compliment from a stranger that made you feel particularly good).

Heck, sometimes I'll drop a post-it in the jar if I've just had a particularly great attitude or outcome of an otherwise normal day ("Full day teaching about health, played with the kids, a shag with the wife and didn't bite my nails!").

At the start of every new year (and sometimes if I'm feeling blue), I open up my jar and look through the post-its to pick me up. Upon reading, I'm recalling those peak moments and remembering my greatness in a flash. It works every time.

It's a great family practice to develop as well. We can celebrate together, individually, and with each other.

However you may choose, the important part is to write down and celebrate life's moments worth remembering. With all the seeming negativity in the world, it's a true gift to recall the joyous moments you've had and shared.

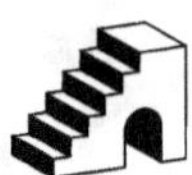

BOTTOM LINE:

- It's crucial to fortify our confidence by writing down the successful moments in daily life we may otherwise forget.

- Simply get a mason jar, some post-its, and a pen to start the practice.

- Do it as a family to share in each other's successes.

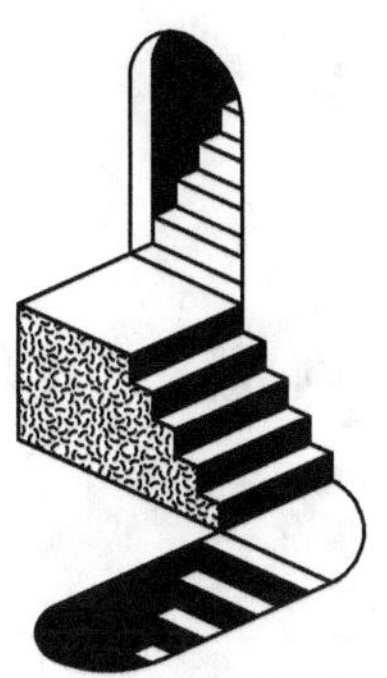

THIRD FLIGHT

Mind your posture

> # A good stance and posture reflect a proper state of mind.
>
> - Morihei Ueshiba

"We've got to take it easy today; my neck is killing me again," Max said with a wince before the start of a training session.

As a vocal performance coach and international entrepreneur, Max spent a lot of time sitting at pianos and desks, most likely unconsciously hunching forward while pecking at keys.

"Sounds bad today. Have you noticed when the pain flares up most?" I asked.

"Sitting at the piano with clients mostly, but certainly at my desk if I'm doing back to back video calls..."

"We've got to do something."

So we made a plan to do a workspace ergonomic check at his home the following week.

When the time came, I had him show me his office and how he was sitting. It was quickly evident what the culprits were:

His desk was too high in relation to his chair height. His keyboard and monitor were too far away. His chair offered no lumbar support.

And because of this, his body was compensating in all sorts of ways—his head jutted forward, his shoulders and mid back rounded, and he had almost no core control to keep his lower back straight.

I smiled, as we had talked about adjusting his workspace for better posture multiple times over the years of coaching together. I guess finally seeing him sit at his sub-optimal desk had me inadvertently flash an "I told you so" dad face.

"Is it that bad?" he sheepishly said.

"Haha you caught me... let's just say I think I can see a few things for us to focus on..."

"I break seated posture into three simple components: push, pull, tilt. As in—push the lower back forward... pull the shoulders back... tilt the chin up. It's an easy three point checklist to see if your posture is aligned."

I also had him order a posture correcting harness—one of my favorite spinal alignment devices to wear when retraining ourselves to sit and stand better.

We corrected what we could for the moment—fitted his posture corrector, ordered a better ergonomic chair, and practiced the push, pull, tilt checklist a few times.

"Push... pull... tilt. Got it. Do you really think this will help my neck?"

"For sure. Give it a couple of weeks to really feel the difference. And hey, pain is the best teacher. If you're out of alignment again you'll know it!"

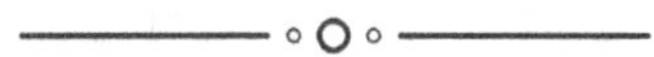

We've heard the terms before—"sitting is the new smoking"... "tech neck."

Buzz words for sure, and there are true, often severe consequences of chronic poor posture. Did you know when in the "tech neck" position (looking down at your phone) the weight of your head increases by up to 500% on your spine?[1] That's like taking the average head weight of 12 lbs and increasing it to 60 lbs! I loathe to think what my big head weighs under those conditions.

Poor posture while seated doesn't fare much better either, with slouching increasing disc pressure by up to 60% and creating significant strain on the spine. Put these issues together and it's no wonder back pain—to which poor posture is a major contributor—costs Americans over $100 billion in medical bills and lost productivity per year.[2]

But the path to healing is rarely surgery. In my opinion, a majority of spinal pain and dysfunction stemming from poor posture can be solved with a few easy steps: optimize the environment, develop awareness, and practice stability.

Environment: Like Max, we've got to make sure our working spaces fit our unique needs.

Awareness: We've got to know what good posture looks and feels like.

Stability: Because modern conveniences such as phones and com-puters have us in the wrong position for hours a day, the necessary musculature we need is often weak and deconditioned! We've got to develop the intrinsic strength to hold our bodies together so that we can maintain the necessary alignment.

Here's how to fix your desk posture in just a few minutes, as recommended by ergonomics expert Olivier Girard:

Chair: Back is approximately 90 degrees to the seat, perhaps with a little give so leaning back lends another 5 degrees. Raise the seat to maximum height, sit in a chair with full butt on the seat cushion and slowly lower the chair until your feet are fully and firmly touching the floor, with no pressure behind the knees. If you don't have an adjustable chair, ideally the seat is 16-20 inches off the floor for those of us in the 5 '2 to 6' 2 height range (including padding of chair), with roughly a 90 degree angle at the knee. Have pronounced lumbar (low back) support, with the greatest amount of support focused just above your belt line.

Desk: Find optimal height by resting your lower wrist area on the corner of the desk—ideally, hands rest flat and comfortably, with no distinct pressure point on wrist or hands. If you can't adjust the desk, raise the chair so you're comfortably aligned and source a foot rest so your feet can once again be flat as before. Usually the keyboard is 22-32 inches from the floor for those in the 5'2 to 6'2 height range.

Computer: Have your monitor set up so the top of the screen is slightly below eye level when sitting up with good posture, screen tilted upward 10 degrees from horizontal (as you would position a book while reading it). Lower monitor 1-2 inches if you wear progressive lenses. The monitor should be about an arm's length away from where you're seated. Ensure text is large enough to read from that distance so you're not leaning forward and squinting to see it!

In addition to Girard's guidance, improved room and screen lighting is critical for posture, too. Chronic exposure to LED and fluorescent overhead bulbs with flickering can cause eye strain and headaches and may contribute to increased risk of eye disease. Research on fluorescent lighting suggests potential links to cataracts, though this remains debated. Ideally, use bulbs with a CRI (color rendering index) of 90 or higher and below 3000 Kelvin on the color temperature scale. Warmer lighting also promotes a calmer vibe throughout the day.[3] I use Iris Tech software to control the monitor's light spectrum, thus controlling glare and adding an orange hue.

Check for yourself right now if reading this at home—does your workspace/home desk meet these criteria?

Environment: Ideally, you've got an adjustable desk and seat that allows for such an array of options, though just making a few of these simple adjustments can yield great benefit along with utilizing the "push-pull-tilt" sequence. Bonus points for creating your car seat with similar conditions and adding some lumbar support!

Awareness: Are you in pain while working at a desk or driving? Your body will surely express discomfort with nagging pain in your head, neck or back if they're out of alignment! Stop, notice the pain, and practice "Push, Pull, Tilt" to achieve the optimal spinal position. Make sure to keep feet facing forward and knees maintaining hip width apart. This will also support hip alignment—crucial for lower body posture.

Stability: This simple, progressive routine helps keep the necessary muscles strong and chronic spinal dysfunction at bay:

Neck extenders: Seated or standing, inhale through the belly while simultaneously pushing head back, giving yourself a slight "double chin." Exhale and bring your head forward. Repeat five to eight times.

Shoulder squeezers: Seated or standing, inhale through the belly while simultaneously pinching shoulder blades together. Hold for a count and allow shoulders to return forward. Repeat five to eight times.

Core activators: Standing, hands on hip bones, exhale all the air in your belly until you feel your core activate (you should feel muscle tightening under your fingertips if placed in the right area). Inhale and release core activation. Repeat five to eight times.

Perform this routine whenever you notice poor posture creeping in. The practice pairs nicely with a five minute work break walk as well!

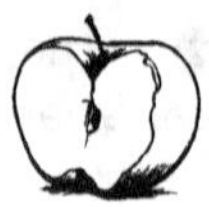

BOTTOM LINE:

- Posture correction can be easy—we've just got to know how to set up and access the right way to sit while working and driving.

- Adjust the work environment first and then practice strengthening your body's proper posture muscles to resolve it for good.

- Purchasing a posture corrector can offer a kickstart to this process and provide an easy reminder of proper body alignment.

Once you've got pure water, make sure it's rich in minerals

> You are comprised of 84
> minerals... you are not living
> on earth. You are earth.
>
> - Aubrey Marcus

"Andy? Andy. I'm Derek. Nice to meet you. Thanks for having us," I said, extending my hand.

"Hey Derek, yes, it's a pleasure to finally meet. Thanks for coming to Oliver's birthday party."

One thing parenting books don't teach you is the art of small talk with other parents at kid birthdays—a skill set all to its own.

Getting five good minutes with a parent before interruptions of tears or something breaking is about all you can hope for.

"Michelle told me your family has a farm up the coast," I continued. "How awesome! I was surrounded by farms growing up. There's something delightfully aromatic about cow manure."

Andy laughed.

"Oh yes, the smells—certain musks only a farmer could love."

"She said you grow citrus, is that right?"

"Correct, navel oranges mostly."

"Awesome. Huge fruit guy over here. I've been following Zach Bush's podcasts about the importance of soil quality to grow food that actually has any nourishment. Big Agriculture is crazy! The synthetic pesticides, monocropping, yielding food devoid of most vitamins and minerals... how did I not know about this until a couple of years ago?"

"It's wild, really," Andy said. "Practices employed 50 years ago like using indiscriminate synthetic pesticides and ammonia-based fertilizers are still being used today on a mass scale. Yet, what was a boon to a growing population back then has essentially killed the inherent life in the soil today."

"Life in the soil," I pondered. "What do you mean? In layman's terms for me, please."

"Well, nutrients are still in the dirt, but there are fungi and bacteria—elements of life that break down soil in ways that make the minerals absorbable into the plant that we eat. Those factors are missing, and that makes the soil effectively dead and thus our food quality diminished."

"I see. So while we're often eating food that looks the same, the quality of it is wildly different depending on how the soil is treated and maintained?"

"Pretty much, yes. Owning a small family farm has me sympathize with why the industry has gotten this way—agricultural margins are slim. But our food supply is contingent on the soil it's grown in."

"Can it be done? Can soil be brought back?" I asked.

"With time, we think so. We've been trying cover cropping methods on a few acres to find out. That's had us use a fraction of the spray and brought back some of the natural ecosystem... snails, butterflies... so that's good. But it's been challenging. The yield is lighter than in the past, so we're still trying to find the right equilibrium."

"Sounds like regenerating soil and the habitat it's in can take years—time many farmers don't think they can survive without."

"Exactly."

Crash *Waaaaaa!*

A ruckus in the playroom stops our conversation in its tracks.

"Excuse me, I've got to check on that."

"Yeah, that sounds like mine. I'll come too."

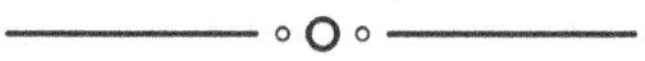

Minerals serve a myriad of benefits to our bodies. We often think of vitamins as crucial micronutrients (which they are), but it is the minerals we consume that serve a host of immunological, neurological, and muscular functions within the body.

A few examples of the roles marvelous minerals play in our health:

Magnesium: Involved in over 400 processes within the body, many of them related to the functioning of our parasympathetic nervous system or the "rest and digest" mode. Also crucial in synthesizing vitamin D into a usable form within our bodies.

Potassium: Essential for muscular contractions, cellular fluid balance, and nerve function.

Calcium: Crucial for bone density, muscular contractions, and blood clotting.

Zinc: Improves immune function, metabolism, and reproductive health.

These are just a few of the major and trace minerals we need to consume regularly for optimal health.

Minerals must be consumed in our diets. Unfortunately, due to the extreme soil degradation Andy spoke about, the minerals we need are found less and less in our standard food supply.

Examples of mineral deficiency include muscle weakness or spasms, brittle hair and nails, skin issues, tingling or numbness, and frequent infections or illness.

Even if you're not experiencing such extremes, a lack of circulating minerals can lead to reduced energy, cognition, sex drive, athletic performance, and increased anxiousness.

This is why supplementing with minerals is often crucial to long term well-being. I could feel a difference almost immediately the first time I added a dose of minerals to my supplement regimen!

There are many options to choose from when searching for ways to increase mineral intake, and I like to boost my mineral intake with liquids, as it promotes better hydration and adds few to no calories.

Here are a few ways I like to get more minerals in:

Au naturel: Squeeze a lemon wedge and drop a pinch of quality Colima, Celtic, or Redmond salts into your first glass of water of the day. This will provide plenty of sodium and potassium—crucial for cellular fluid balance and peristalsis (intestinal movement to help you "go" in the morning).

Supplement: I personally squirt a dash of Trace Minerals into my first water bottle.

Scoop: Use a serving of Irish or sea moss gel in your smoothie or drink of choice. This path also has the added benefit of extra vitamins and antioxidants.

Almost anytime is a fine time to increase mineral intake throughout the day, and I prefer to consume mine first thing in the morning. I feel it helps me hydrate, especially when my body is craving water intake after a long night's rest.

If you're anything like me, you'll feel the added benefit of supercharging your water almost right away!

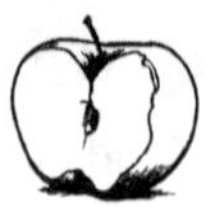

BOTTOM LINE:

- Minerals serve thousands of functions within our body and brain.

- Due to soil depletion in mainstream agriculture, there has been a large reduction in mineral quantities within our food supply.

- Adding a mineral supplement to our clean water or smoothie is an easy way to improve digestion, organ health, neurotransmitter activity, stress, and much more.

- We lose up to a liter of water through breathing every night—replenish your liquid and mineral stores every morning!

Five or more servings of fruits and vegetables per day

> **We should all be eating fruits and vegetables as if our lives depend on it - because they do.**
>
> - Michael Greger

"**W**ell Claudette, we got your labs back," said Dr. Meg. "Based on HbA1c results, you're newly diagnosed as a type 2 diabetic. On top of that, your cholesterol and triglycerides are high. I would like to spend some time reviewing this information and discuss ways to support your health."

Claudette was silent. Her father died of complications with diabetes. She knew what was at stake.

"Your previous doctor said you were resistant to taking medication to manage symptoms, is that correct?"

"Yes, my father experienced massive complications from medications, and it is not something I would like to consider at this time. I would like to try other options if possible before I would further consider."

"I see," Dr. Meg said—she was a smart resident not to force the issue. Other more experienced doctors had tried to, unsuccessfully. Dr. Meg had created a therapeutic relationship with the patient. She reviewed the guidelines and more conventional allopathic recommendations with Claudette but was also open to working with her to achieve their goals in another way.

"Well, there are ways that we could work to lower your blood sugar and other at-risk markers. Has anyone on your medical team spoken with you about making some diet and lifestyle changes yet?"

"No, not really..." Claudette responded.

Dr. Meg went on.

"Perhaps we could start by talking about food as medicine. Positive nutrition choices, ones in which we prioritize eating fruits or vegetables or a more whole-food, plant-based diet, have been shown to have a profound effect on well-being and lowering metabolic risk factors. If you're truly serious about making changes without medication, this is where we would begin. Small changes eventually make big changes, and we will work together."

Claudette began to see food as an opportunity to improve her health.

"Okay... I'll do it. I'm in. How do we start?"

Claudette got serious about her diet: fruits and vegetables became the foundation, and she stopped stress-snacking on processed food. Nine months later? Her HbA1c was below 6.5 (no longer diabetic), and her triglycerides were under 100. She also felt better energy, more stable mood, and was sleeping better. She felt motivated to continue to make substantial changes to support her health.

"I was thrilled for her," Dr. Meg said. "She was able to not only improve her objective lab markers but also improve her quality of life just by making healthier food selections and relating to food as her medicine. That's what integrative health is all about."

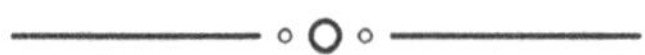

Fruits and vegetables should be the foundation of nearly all diets.

Regardless of whatever food pyramid the government is pushing, you can rarely go wrong when making fruits and vegetables the foundation of your diet.

No foods nourish the body more than plants. Fruits and vegetables contain cancer-fighting phytonutrients, antioxidants, vitamins, and minerals that keep us feeling our best. Increasing fruit and vegetable consumption may sound like run-of-the-mill advice, but consider this: a 2007-2010 national survey found 60% of children don't eat enough fruits, and 93% of children don't consume enough vegetables to meet their minimal daily requirements.[4]

After 15 years of health coaching experience, I'd assert adults are no different.

I used to say people should consume seven to nine servings of fruits and vegetables per day, if possible local, organic, and ripe. While I still think that a noble aim, just getting a consistent five is more than enough for the busy parent and business person getting just one or two!

When starting with clients, I make fruit and vegetable intake the priority above calories ("Count carrots, not calories," I quip). They're easier to track and have a more positive impact on the psyche for most people.

Here are a few ways to boost intake if you find it hard to increase fruit and veggie count:

- In a smoothie

- Choosing your staple/favorite variety and making it part of a daily habit

- Making enough vegetables at dinner for lunch the next day

- In supplement form by way of powder or capsule

- Start your grocery shopping ventures in the produce section

As ever, not all produce is created equal. Beware of the pesticides, herbicides and fungicides sprayed on conventional (non-organic) produce. Pest sprays have been proven to promote non-Hodgkin's lymphoma in regular users. In addition, a $10 billion settlement was reached with users of RoundUp (the most common weed killer used in mainstream agriculture) who alleged the company failed to warn about the cancer risks associated with the product.[5]

Check out the Environmental Working Group's annual Dirty Dozen and Clean Fifteen produce lists to determine if buying organic would be a better choice for the variety you eat. Overall, it's advised to buy organic when able.

Whichever you choose, wash your produce in a 4:1 mix of water and apple cider vinegar (ACV). The ACV solution helps remove bacteria and some pesticide residue better than water alone.

I won't say this extra step is a must because many people aren't eating any produce in the first place (don't throw the baby out with the vinegar-soaked bath water, you dig?) but US foods are fraught with chemicals that could be doing unknown harm to your digestive tract, so it may be worth the extra time.

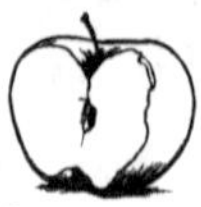

BOTTOM LINE:

- "Let food be thy medicine"—perhaps the wisest quote of all.

- Harnessing produce as a cornerstone of your diet is the fastest way to get healthier, leaner, and longer-lived.

- "Count carrots, not calories."

- There are all sorts of ways to prepare produce and boost intake if you're not naturally inclined to its taste.

Note: *Nothing is a panacea, not even fresh, local, organic produce. Some vegetables are hard to digest (cruciferous ones such as broccoli, cabbage, and Brussels sprouts)... Salad greens can wreak havoc on someone with IBS... Strawberries/fruits with seeds are brutal for those with Crohn's disease. That being said, there's a fruit or vegetable for nearly everyone, and they hold nutritional benefits we won't find in any other food group, so it's worth doing your due diligence to find the ones that fit your taste and biological individuality.*

Get curious about your gut health and food sensitivities

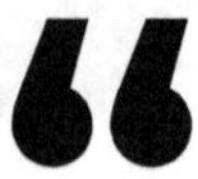

The road to health is paved with good intestines!

- Sherry A. Rogers

"But... that's how I've always done it. Work. Come home. A huge bowl of cereal."

I was on the defensive. Wifey had just questioned my after-work snack habit.

"Yes, but do you think another after-work snack would suffice? Sophie is getting into the habit of wanting a bowl of junky cereal when she sees you have one, and I'd really like to keep her afternoon sweets to a minimum."

"But... but... but!"

"And you're so gassy after eating cereal, too!" she added.

Called out for flatulence—a dagger through the heart and stomach.

Hi, I'm Derek—recovering junky cereal addict. Growing up I would bookend my school days with a hearty bowl or two of Froot Loops for breakfast and a well-earned snack of them upon returning home.

I must've gone through two boxes per week myself.

The satisfaction of cold milk (2%!) coupled with sweet, crunchy cereal had me hooked. Nearly any flavor would do:

Cap'n Crunch (peanut butter protein!)

Honey Bunches of Oats (a "healthier" approach)

Froot Loops (for a morning fruit infusion)

Count Chocula (because who doesn't need marshmallows as a part of balanced morning nourishment?)

Sugar Smacks (ok, ok, I can't even fake this one—it's blissful abomination)

While my youthful metabolism and activity level could handle the empty calories, I didn't get the true impact until many years later.

You see... most of my life I've had persistent gas. It was legitimately embarrassing. Friends would mock me at sleepovers. My college roommate would admonish me for smoking him out in our dorm room. My wife (and later daughter) would bemoan "Daddyyyy" for my smelly indiscretions in the living room.

Much as I tried to do it when I was alone, the smell would linger long enough for someone to walk into the room and call me out!

I can laugh about it now, and I know it wasn't pleasant for my family and friends to be around. But honestly? It was physically uncomfortable for me too. The bloating and gas pressure were so intense I'd have to fart or I'd burst!

Funny or not, no one wants to be "that guy." But I was.

And since I'd had that experience for as long as I could remember, I surrendered to the belief that occasional smelly gas is just my lot in life… something that just "is," and there's nothing else I can do about it…

It took me until I was 34 years old (all the while eating cereal) and studying for a new integrative health coaching certification to begin to see this gas issue was something I could actually do something about.

Fast forward a few months into my integrative health studies and personal wellness discovery, I decided to perform a battery of digestive tests and see how my insides were functioning at a cellular level. It would be good practice to work with the instructor on how to interpret them for myself at first and then learn to guide others.

Upon testing my gut health, it was clear to the instructor reading my labs that overall my gut health was excellent, and I had one very clear culprit in my digestive issue.

"Derek, as you can see on this line of your food Intolerance test, you've got a high amount of Candida Albicans—a naturally occurring fungus found in our bodies that can become overgrown and problematic, leading to a host of mild to moderate effects. Have you noticed any digestive discomfort in any scenarios? Say, after eating a processed snack like crackers or cereal?"

I was nailed.

"Yeah, you could say that," I sheepishly replied.

While a small amount of candida in our digestive tract is common and not typically something to worry about, over time it can compromise our delicate microbiome and run rampant in a body in the presence of high sugar and yeast consumption. (Read: junky cereals.) "Symptoms include chronic fatigue, brain fog, bloating, and gas."

Oye.

It suddenly made so much sense. All these years of eating sugary cereal (among other offenders like cookies and crackers)—I'd been literally feeding the problem this whole time.

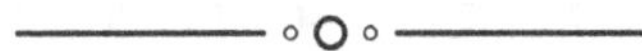

It can be so easy to fall into and stay in a grooved routine, especially if there's a payoff like comfort food, procrastination/avoidance, or distraction.

Routines are comforting to the brain, but there is a cost. The more frequently we do them, the less we become aware of their impact.

When the trigger happens—for me, walking in after work—the brain's habit circuits (basal ganglia and neocortex) kick in, pushing me to go through the routine and get that reward (the sweet, crunchy, satisfying cereal).

Interrupting it begins with stepping outside of ourselves for a moment and looking at our patterns.

Consider yours:

- What are the triggers, cues, first "dominoes" that lead to overeating, drinking, bingeing?

- Is there a cost to the behavior you want to stop paying for?

- What would it take for you to circumvent the habit?

- What would be the reward of changing?

- Do you need support or to get in partnership with someone to help you stay accountable?

I asked my wife not to buy cereal anymore—no boxes in the house, period—and to call me out if I caved and bought one myself. Because I knew one box would lead to another, and another, until I was right back where I started.

Now it's pretty straightforward: When I cut out cereal and processed foods, my gas goes away. If I eat cereal and processed foods, my gas comes back.

I'm proud of myself for this discovery. What began as a decades-long unconscious routine had real consequences I didn't want to live with anymore. Without support to uncover the root cause of my embarrassing gas, I'd probably still be throwing up my hands and accepting it as inevitable.

In the words of Maya Angelou: "People are afraid to be pried loose from their ignorance because they know their ignorance so well..."

Make no mistake—many days I still experience the temptation to have a bowl of cereal... I just feel and smell a whole lot better without it.

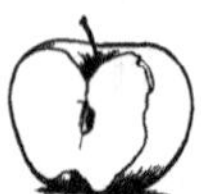

BOTTOM LINE:

- To save energy our brains are wired to repeat actions without thinking about them—especially when there is a reward involved.

- Questioning and interrupting the routines that negatively impact our lives is the start of beginning new, positive ones.

- Food sensitivities and gut imbalances (like candida overgrowth) can cause uncomfortable symptoms that we might just accept as "normal"—but they're not!

- Consider testing for food sensitivities if you have persistent digestive issues, fatigue, or other unexplained symptoms.

Set up your sleep space

> **If you want to change the world, start off by making your bed.**
>
> - Admiral William H. McRaven

I hadn't been sleeping well.

In Summer 2018, we moved into a home which had an eastern facing bay window that got early sunshine. The home was in a more urban area of Los Angeles as well, so the street lights were always on.

It also stayed hotter for longer, leaving me tossing and turning unless I turned on the air (which at LA utility prices, this dad didn't want to do).

"What the hell is going on? I slept great in our last place. Now I feel like I'm tossing and turning every night," I complained to my visiting mother-in-law one morning.

That evening she came into our vacant bedroom to grab something for our daughter.

"No wonder you're not sleeping—your curtains aren't blocking any light! It's practically daytime in here."

"Oh, I guess I hadn't thought of that," I said, sheepishly after she pointed to the obvious.

Don't you hate when your mother-in-law is right?!

We ordered a set of blackout curtains that night. Couple those with a new, big room fan (because my ass still isn't paying for AC), and I was back to sleeping much better soon thereafter.

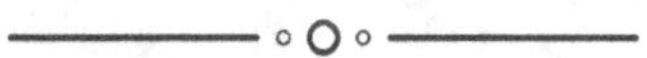

Setting up a proper sleep space matters. A lot. It's especially crucial as we age and quality sleep is no longer a given. Take it from a guy who uses a sleep tracker because he was doing it all wrong for a long time.

Here are my bedroom must-haves if I'm going to sleep like a champ:

Use soft, red-spectrum lighting: Light bulbs with red or amber hues have minimal impact on melatonin suppression, helping you fall asleep faster than blue and white light from standard bulbs. Since incandescent bulbs are no longer available in the US, opt for high-quality red or amber LED bulbs for bedroom lighting. Avoid cheap LEDs, which often flicker (even imperceptibly) and can increase sleep latency.

No TV in the bedroom: The blue light from the screen and stimulus from content is a double whammy of sleep latency and restlessness for me.

Make the room as dark as possible: This may be most important of all. Melatonin is one of our main hormones responsible for sleep. It is most abundantly released by the brain's pineal gland after light signals stop coming into the eyes' Suprachiasmatic Nucleus (SCN) which acts as the body's internal clock, regulating when we're up and when we're to sleep. A bedroom devoid of any light cues the SCN to promote sleep by triggering melatonin production and suppressing brain activity associated with wakefulness.[6]

Darkness is the primary access to begin this cascade. Use blackout curtains, put towels under doors to block hallway light, cover up thermostats and other glowing or light-emitting devices. The darker the better.

Cooler room temperatures: As we fall asleep, our body's natural circadian rhythm lowers our core temperature—this helps us attain essential phases of restorative sleep. Warmer room temperatures can prevent our bodies from achieving the necessary internal temperature reduction, pull us out of these deeper sleep levels, and even wake us up! Cooler temperatures also encourage further release of melatonin—a 1-2 punch. Aim for a room temperature of 62-67 degrees. To this end, I'm a proponent of sleeping in the nude with just a pair of comfy socks on.

Fall asleep to white noise: White noise is defined as a random signal with equal intensity across various frequencies. This creates the characteristic "hissing" sound that can mask disruptive environmental noises and help promote sleep.[7] In layman's terms, think of the sound that radio static, a fan, or air conditioner makes. White noise helps sleep onset by masking background sounds that might otherwise wake us up or make it hard to fall asleep (like traffic, dogs barking, or a partner snoring). The steady, predictable sound can be soothing and help your mind settle, reducing racing thoughts or anxiety. Some people prefer alternatives like pink noise (lower, more natural sounding) or brown noise (deeper and even more mellow). There are many apps to choose from, but to me nothing beats an oscillating floor fan pointed at my bed. This one gets bonus points for cooling down the room temperature as well!

Clean air in the bedroom: Americans spend approximately 87% of their time indoors and another 5.5% inside vehicles, meaning we spend about 93% of our lives in enclosed spaces. This lack of outdoor exposure affects circadian rhythm regulation, vitamin D production, and overall health.[8] What's more, the majority of pollutants we inhale actually come from within our home! Mold, dust, volatile organic compounds from furniture, paint, or cleaning products can all be at play unconsciously impacting our health. When we sleep, we breathe 7,000-8,000 times. Make sure that the air you're breathing during that time is as clean as possible! Certain house plants can do a great job of removing specific household toxins like formaldehyde and benzene, but we lean on an air purifier to remove a broader range of offenders. Plus, it gets extra credit for the white noise it creates.

Unplug electronics and routers (or at least keep them out of your room): Beyond the light they give off, (which messes with your darkness), there's some debate about whether electromagnetic fields from devices affect sleep. The research is all over the place and nobody's quite sure how it would work. What we do know? Blue light from screens tanks your melatonin production. That's not up for debate. Some people swear they're sensitive to electromagnetic fields and can't sleep with a router nearby. Thing is, when researchers test this in controlled settings where people don't know if the device is on or off, the connection falls apart. But here's the bottom line: get the electronics out of your bedroom anyway. Your sleep will thank you.[9]

Turn off or keep phone as far away from you as possible: In addition to releasing EMFs (as above), incoming alerts turn on your phone's screen, releasing blue light into a dark room. This can interrupt deep sleep (even if you don't necessarily wake up from it). If you must keep the phone nearby, turn off its WiFi, be sure to minimize screen brightness, cover it with a t-shirt, and set the device to "silent" mode, thus minimizing disturbances.

Read: I love to read before bed. It lowers my stress levels by shifting focus away from worries and onto the page, slowly lulling me to sleep. Studies show reading can reduce stress by up to 68%, even more than listening to music or going for an evening walk.[10] To this end, reading cues your brain to transition from the busy pace of the day into a slower rhythm, quieting racing thoughts that often interfere with falling asleep. Pick something calming—skip suspense, horror, or anything too mentally stimulating. Keep the room light soft and warm (as noted in the environment point above), and choose printed books or e-readers with no blue light emissions. I know once I start to sleepily drop the book on my face, it's time for lights out!

Use appropriate mattress, clean, comfy sheets and pillow: These are essential for ergonomics, or "the design of things for their safe, efficient and comfortable use." Appropriate bed and pillow density can help us wake up feeling youthful and refreshed or achy and slow. We're in virtually the same position for 7-9 hours—better make sure that what we're resting on for that time makes us feel good upon waking up! Sleeping on regularly washed, breathable sheets keeps the dust mites away and our core body temperature cool.

Vacuum your mattress a few times per year: Yes, it's strange. But stranger still is the amount of dead skin you'll pick up in the process. We're constantly shedding dermis, and some of it falls through our porous sheet material. Dust mites feed primarily on our dead skin(!), so suck them and their "food" off of your bed and be amazed how your allergies and breathing clear up!

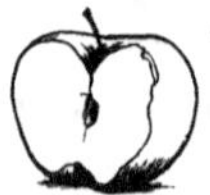

BOTTOM LINE:

- Sleep quality and quantity are greatly influenced by our bedroom's environment.

- Your senses should be at total ease—manage touch, light, sound, smell and temperature in the sleep space to achieve optimal resting conditions.

- Do a bedroom "audit" and see how many of these suggestions you can implement tonight. I can near-guarantee you'll wake up feeling more refreshed because of the changes!

- Visit **www.eattheapplebook.com** to get your downloadable restless checklist so you can sleep better tonight.

Make a healthier unhealthy choice

> # Never take the entire snack bag to the couch.
>
> - Derek Opperman

"I don't care what you try to convince me of, I'm not giving up my Oreos," Terry said, digging her proverbial heels in on our introductory health coaching call. Terry was part of a corporate wellness challenge I ran with a sales team.

"I'm up for this challenge my boss is having us do, but I like my sweets and don't want to change that…

I also want to lose 10 pounds, so figure that out."

Terry was great. A real southern firecracker with a great sense of humor.

"Okay got it, Terry. What I'm hearing you say is you'd like to see some fat loss but don't want to eat like a rabbit to do so, is that correct?"

"Bingo."

"Let's talk about portion sizes: how many Oreos or cookies do you have per day?"

"Oh, four or five."

"Got it. For this challenge, are you open to eating one to three, walking away from the bag and seeing if you're satisfied with a couple less cookies?"

"Oh. Uh… okay."

I think Terry anticipated more of a fight from me.

"You see, Terry, we don't need to give up everything tasty in the name of a trimmer waistline. Sometimes we just need to consume a little less, and that yields a great benefit without playing a zero sum game. Each cookie has 75-100 calories. If you eat 2-3 less per day, we're saving 150-300 calories per day, 1,000-2,000 calories per week, 4,000-8,000 calories per month, 50,000-100,000 calories per year."

"Oh wow… never thought of it like that."

"Right?! Just let me send you my favorite vegan date ball recipe and then we'll really be cooki…"

"Easy there, buddy." She cut me off with a wink.

Over the next five weeks, Terry ended up losing those 10 lbs by eating two fewer cookies, going on an evening walk (which was another negotiation), and adding 1-2 servings of fruits and veggies per day (often canned because she didn't like to cook). Nothing fancy or drastic. Just a little less of some things, a little more of others.

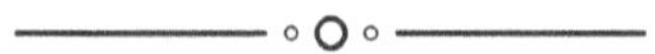

Terry's story is the kind of success I'm most proud of. Awesome results on her own terms, just a few subtle changes done consistently—especially impressive when you consider how easy it is to eat empty calories these days. We're practically encouraged to. Portions are larger. Our favorite foods are more accessible than ever. And healthier options? Buried behind the junk.

With endless convenience at our fingertips, it's easy to mindlessly default to processed crap. I've been coaching for 15 years, and I've seen the same patterns repeat: people defend keeping comfort foods around because they're familiar, they feel good, they're easy. Or they try going cold turkey and can't handle the pull. The foods always win.

And I get it—a midday snack feels good. Dessert after dinner feels good. A beer after work feels good.

I like all of those things, too!

But like the philosopher Paracelsus said, "The dose makes the poison."

You can still enjoy comfort foods. Just have less of them. In my experience, that's how you hit your goals without going insane.

Check out a few of these swaps:

A bowl of oatmeal or yogurt with toppings for a bowl of sweet, generic cereal (this one is for me).

Half-sweetened iced tea for regular sweet tea.

Half cauliflower rice, half white rice.

Americano coffee with half & half and two sugars instead of a latte and six sugars (the standard amount major coffee chains mix into your beverage).

Simply do a web search of "healthy/homemade swaps for *enter food*"—you'll find higher quality pre-made options and recipes to try. And of course you can always split a burger and fries and an entree-sized salad with a fellow diner.

For the most part, our bodies are adept at consuming too much food once in a while. In fact, a lot of research points to the benefit of occasional feast-worthy meals for hormone regulation, satiety, and mental health. Simply resisting temptation for too long doesn't work for anyone, and we'll always ultimately rebound in spite of our best intentions.

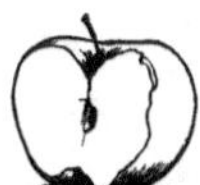

BOTTOM LINE:

- You can have your cake and eat it, too—just a smaller slice.

- Zero-sum games are hard to stick with. Look for healthier swaps, recipes, and plate shares to satisfy cravings on better terms.

- Step away from the bag, plate, or pint after a couple of bites—you can't eat what's out of reach.

- Brush your teeth after your portion—it's the ultimate craver tamer!

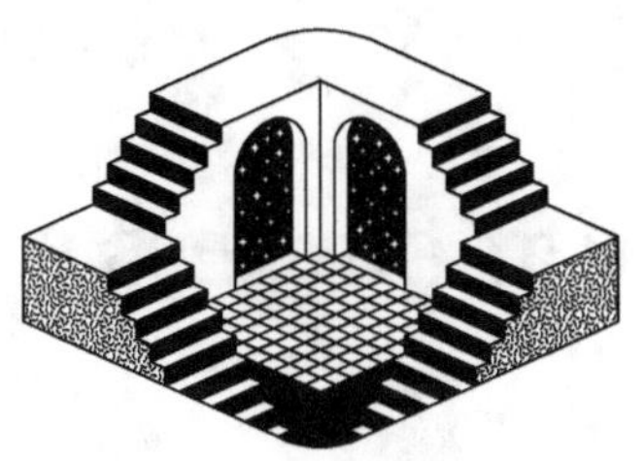

FOURTH FLIGHT

Eat out less

Hey, I wanna lose weight. Let's go out to restaurants more often.

- No one, ever

"I am a mess. I've never been so heavy in my life," Sean said, as he broke down to me while warming up on the treadmill.

Due to a high stress job, supporting his elderly mother, and a relationship that was breaking down, he had not been in a good place for months.

"I am over 30 pounds above my goal weight, and I just don't know what to do."

"Okay," I said in a calming voice. "Let's talk this out. Let's have a look at your current eating practices and see what's there to start."

"Well I haven't been eating that unhealthily, but I have been eating out a lot. Or ordering delivery to my house."

"Ah! Our first clue… say more about your restaurant habit," I said.

"Yeah, I've just been so busy that I haven't had any time to cook, so I just order something and have it sent to me."

"Okay, got it, and how frequently would that be, on average?"

"Probably two or three meals per day… sometimes snacks too."

I stared blankly at him and he slowly, sheepishly smiled.

"I know. I know I've got to get a handle on this."

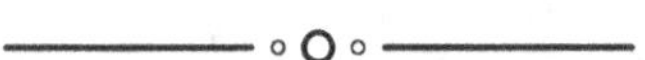

Sean's case is not extraordinary or unique. When life gets too busy with work, family, and social obligations, food prep is one of the first things to go. After all, cooking—especially for one person—feels like a lot of work. The grocery shopping, the meal prep, the cooking, the cleanup. Compare that to Uber Eats: tap your phone, food shows up, eat it, toss the container. Done.

Beyond the convenience, eating out or ordering in comes with a few steep costs.

First, the literal dollars and cents of eating out is upwards of five to six times the cost of preparing the same meal for yourself. My family of four cannot seem to spend less than $100 going out to a restaurant, (not including alcohol), so the cost savings alone may be worth the price of cooking at home.

Beyond monetary price, the health costs are what we ought to look at here. According to a study by the University of Michigan, families who cook at home more frequently have a statistically higher Healthy Eating Index, a USDA guideline that measures the quality of foods consumed in accordance with Dietary Guidelines for Americans.[1]

Think about it: restaurants make their money by serving up a meal that is delicious and satisfying and has us coming back again and again. Do you know what is delicious and satisfying to our brain and tastebuds?

Salt, fat, sugar, carbohydrates—ingredients your conventional restaurant kitchen will use liberally to have you saying, "Now that was a good meal!"

Granted, many restaurants are finding their niche by choosing healthier ingredients with more balanced proportions, but I would assert that the majority do not abide by the same standard.

My own anecdotal observations are that many restaurants are stingy with protein, quality fats, and vegetable servings—the cornerstone of an actual healthy diet.

Restaurants are also notorious for using seed oils that are highly inflammatory to our bodies. Oils are one of the more expensive line items in the kitchen, so restaurant owners are apt to save on cost and use a cheaper option.

When dining out, alcohol and dessert are always tempting. Plus, you have zero control over what the chef cooks with or how much they're going to serve you.

When setting up wellness programs for my clients, I stress the fact that eating out should be special, not a staple. I suggest dining out three times or less per week.

If your lifestyle lends itself to eating out with more frequency than that, here are a few suggestions to make a healthier choice when at the restaurant:

Number one: Ask what oil they cook their food in (pretend you have an allergy and need to know—liability always gets their attention).

Number two: Request a double portion of protein.

Number three: Opt for just one starch on the plate. If you're at a burger joint, choose a hamburger bun and a side salad or a hamburger, protein-style, with a lettuce wrap and the french fries instead.

Number four: Whenever possible, look ahead on Google or Yelp at the restaurant menu. That way, you'll be prepared to know what to order, creating a higher likelihood of making a healthy choice

Number five: Don't drink your calories! That includes alcohol and non. Instead, drink water with lemon, as the lemon will help boost digestion before partaking.

The same principles apply if you tend to order in like Sean (DoorDash, Uber Eats, etc). Give yourself the time to review your options, make adjustments to orders, and prepare your digestive tract with lemon water and some pre-meal movement.

Sean's story has a happy ending: he deleted all of the restaurant delivery service apps from his phone, signed up for a healthy meal delivery service instead, and lost the 30 lbs that were weighing him down. He also saved over $1,000 per month making the switch. More money in his pockets, less waist in his pants—a happy trade I'd make any day!

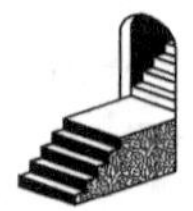

BOTTOM LINE:

- Conscious cooking at home makes a lot of health and financial sense.

- There's arguably nothing more important to health than the food choices one makes on a regular basis.

- Restaurant food is not the way to achieve the body of your dreams—make it special, not a staple.

Be a label reader

> **What the large print giveth, the fine print taketh away.**
>
> - Unknown

"Okay, uh... where do we begin?" Billy asked nervously as we grabbed our shopping carts.

I do grocery store tours with my health coaching clients. It's essential to see their baseline knowledge of how to properly navigate a grocery store in the beginning of a coaching program. Food choices are foundational to their success.

Billy was a relatively healthy guy and was looking to take his physique to the next level. Going from 20% body fat down to 12% is a pretty big step, and since he was getting married in a year he wanted to look as good as possible on the big day.

In order to achieve that lofty goal, we were going to have to get serious about his food regimen. Contrary to popular belief, abs are not made in the kitchen, but before that in the grocery store.

I've found that grocery store tours work best when the client leads me to the foods they typically like and together we either approve the food or find a healthier, reasonable substitute for it.

"Let's start with proteins—what do you typically pick out?" I said.

"I'm a huge fan of barbecue. I could eat that every day," Billy replied. "So we'll usually get some pre-made barbecue pulled pork, chicken, or beef to save time."

"Great," I said. "Show me which brand you like?"

Billy located his pre-made selection of choice and handed the package to me proudly. "What do you think?" he asked with equal parts excitement and nerves.

"Let's have a look and see what the label says," I replied.

Gulp.

It was pretty clear that Billy hadn't considered there may be more to his choice than just shredded pork.

"After pork, the next ingredients are sugar, apple cider vinegar, brown sugar, and molasses."

"Whoa, aren't almost all of those ingredients sugar?" Billy asked.

"Yep, pretty much."

"But wait, it says there's only 7 grams of sugar per serving. That's not so bad, right?"

"On the surface, it would seem that way, but look at the serving size—1/4 cup or 2 ounces, which is only one third to one quarter of a typical serving size. Consume a standard 6-8 ounces and you'd actually be consuming 21 to 28 grams of sugar. It is amazing how food companies will manipulate the label to get you to think you're making a healthier choice than is actually so."

"Yeah. Wow. I guess that barbecue goodness comes at quite a price huh?"

"Buddy, we are just scratching the surface."

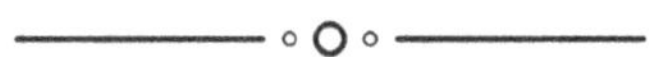

Not to sound like a jaded health professional, but much of the food found in grocery stores isn't healthy. In a capitalistic society, it is profits not food quality that run the economy.

Major food conglomerates dictate what makes it onto the shelves by determining what is addictively tasty and of the best margins... not what is sustaining and nourishing.

Food companies need products that are shelf stable (often not requiring refrigeration), that can satisfy our sweet or salty tooth, and will have us come back for another package next week.

Couple irresistible, lab-designed flavor profiles with deceptive marketing and packaging tactics, and we are often left with food that is high in sugar, inflammatory fats, and calories, and devoid of nutrients.

Oftentimes we are tricked into believing we are making healthy choices when in fact, we are not.

For instance, check out this list of *some* possible names for sugar on a nutrient facts label that are not listed specifically as sugar:

Glucose, Fructose, Corn Syrup, High Fructose Corn Syrup, Corn Syrup Solids, Rice Syrup, Dextrose/Dextrin, Maltose, Lactose, Galactose, Molasses, Caramel. All in all, there are over 60 types of sugar variants food producers use to add to your food![2]

Just as deceptive, look at all the names for highly inflammatory seed oils:

Canola, Corn, Soybean, Cottonseed, Sunflower, Safflower, Rapeseed, Peanut.

Yikes!

Food companies are well aware that the products they're marketing are not healthy, so they must do something so as to have their products look more benign than they actually are.

Check out this serving size for a name brand pickle company: 1/4 pickle.

Nearly one fifth of your sodium intake for the day in a quarter of a pickle... who eats a quarter of a pickle!?

Nutrition Facts

About 4.5 servings per container

Serving Size 1 oz (28g/about ¼ pickle)

Amount Per Serving

Calories 0

	% Daily Value*
Total Fat 0g	0%
Sodium 370mg	16%
Total Carbohydrate 0g	0%
Dietary Fiber 0g	0%
Total Sugars 0g	
Protein 0g	
Calcium 30mg	2%
Potassium 10mg	0%

Not a significant source of saturated fat, trans fat, cholesterol, added sugars, vitamin D, and iron.

*The % Daily Value (DV) tells you how much a nutrient in a serving of food contributes to a daily diet. 2,000 calories a day is used for general nutrition advice.

INGREDIENTS: CUCUMBER, WATER, SALT, VINEGAR, CALCIUM CHLORIDE, NATURAL FLAVORING, SODIUM BENZOATE AND POTASSIUM SORBATE (TO PREVENT SPOILAGE) AND YELLOW 5.

All this to say, we've got to be keenly aware of the food we choose while shopping.

Here are a few things I look out for when shopping for my family and working with clients:

Look for as few ingredients as possible: Ideally, the majority of your shopping cart has single-ingredient choices (i.e., an apple, ground turkey, cinnamon, potato, etc.)

If you can't pronounce the ingredients, you probably shouldn't eat too much of it: Whole foods rarely contain x's and z's in their name, if you know what I mean.

Check the size per serving: As mentioned, this is a prime manipulation zone. A more important consideration is, "How much of this food will you actually eat?"

Check the percent daily value: This paired with serving size tells a lot about how much the food producer is trying to hide from potential purchasers.

Be on the lookout for higher fiber, higher protein, and "excellent source of —" as markers for indicating a better choice.

Check the amount of sugar: Aim for 10 grams or less per serving with most foods.

Look out for the term "enriched with": This typically means a food is so processed that the food company must put vitamins and minerals back into the product. (Look for this in many cereals and breads.)

Look out for artificial dyes: Red 3, Yellow 5 (Tartrazine), and Blue 1 (Brilliant Blue) are petroleum-based products that have been shown to cause allergic reactions, hyperactivity in children, and potential carcinogenic effects at high doses.[3] As of January 2025, these dyes are banned in the United States following an FDA rulemaking process.[4]

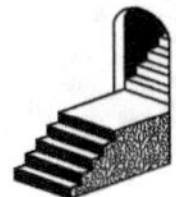

BOTTOM LINE:

- Food companies exist to make a profit first, distributing a healthy or healthier product second (sometimes a distant second).

- Be leery of misleading serving sizes, alternatively labeled sugars, and seed oils—they come in many names.

- When available, refer to the "% daily value" as a better metric of nutrition information (though it's not listed for all items, including sugar).

- Seek ingredients you can easily pronounce.

- In general, the fewer ingredients, the better!

Eat dinner as early as possible

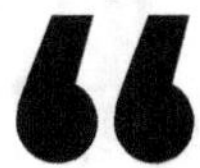

To eat is a necessity, but to eat intelligently is an art.

- Francois de Rochefoucauld

"Derek, you've got to put on some size if you want to compete at the next physique show," said Tim, my second physique coach. I had placed fourth in the last show, and while I was more defined than anyone on the stage, I was also at least 10 pounds of muscle lighter than anyone, too.

"To get your anabolism up, we're going to have you add a meal of oats and whey protein powder before bed."

So eat oats and whey I did. While adding yet another meal to my regimen no doubt increased my weight, shortly after the dietary change I found myself tossing and turning in bed more than ever before. Up to that point I never had an issue falling and staying asleep.

"What the hell is going on?" I wondered as I lay awake, stomach churning...

Now, I know most of you aren't prepping for physique competitions, but this experience taught me something that applies to everyone...

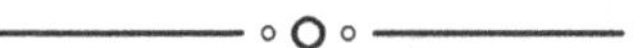

Eating an early dinner is one of the most underrated and under-utilized health hacks we can commit to, especially for those who want to lose weight and sleep better.

Eating dinner (and all other subsequent snacks!) two or more hours away from bedtime holds multiple benefits.

First, it helps increase the quality and quantity of sleep. Did you know that about 10% of the calories you eat get burned just digesting your food? That's called the thermic effect of food—your body has to work to break down what you eat. Protein takes the most work (about 30% of protein calories go toward digestion), carbs are in the middle (5-10%), and fat barely requires any effort (0-3%). When you eat right before bed, your body's busy digesting instead of focusing on the restorative work sleep is supposed to handle.

Studies show that eating within a couple hours of bedtime more than doubles your chances of waking up in the middle of the night. Your metabolism slows down at night, digestion becomes less efficient, and lying down after eating increases your risk of acid reflux and heartburn—all of which mess with your sleep quality. Give yourself at least 2-4 hours between your last meal and bedtime to let your body properly process food before it shifts into sleep mode.[5]

When we give our body ample time between dinner and bed, we're allowing our body to pass the food (at this point called "chyme") on to the small intestine for processing and allowing our liver to focus on detoxification.

We cannot achieve optimal resting states while simultaneously digesting a meal.

According to Ayurveda, our digestive capabilities are strongest between 11 AM and 2 PM,[6] so ideally our biggest meal is around lunchtime. I understand that culturally this can be hard to do. However, whenever able, aim to create the habit of eating your dinners as far away from bed as possible.

If you do eat late, start with a smaller portion, wait 20 minutes, and see if you're still hungry before going back for seconds. Using a smaller plate helps—we tend to fill whatever size plate we're given, so a smaller plate naturally means less food. Smaller plate circumferences equate to smaller portions.

When tracking my sleep, I've noted a nearly 10% decrease in sleep quality (as measured by heart rate variability, resting heart rate, deep sleep, and REM sleep)—all as a result of how much I eat and how late I eat dinner.

Next, eating early is excellent for those looking to lose body fat, as we are typically at our least active in the evenings. Watching shows, lounging with the family are both fine and relaxing rituals, however this abundance of food and lack of movement costs our waistlines dearly.

Eating earlier also gives us ample time to add a little more movement after the meal. Take a leisurely sunset walk after dinner (even if for five minutes), walk about the kitchen and house to prepare for the next day, play with kids or pets—all can help flatten blood sugar spikes much more than sitting still and vegging out.

Brush and floss a few minutes after dinner so you're less tempted to have a late night snack.

When we put time and movement between dinner and bed and then actually rest before sleep, our body finishes digesting, blood sugar stabilizes, and we're primed for quality sleep. With that quality sleep, our body burns more body fat, we make better food choices the next day, and we perform at a higher level in everything we do.

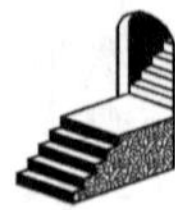

BOTTOM LINE:

- Eat like a prince in the morning, a king in the afternoon, and a pauper at night!

- Your rest and waistline will improve in short order.

Track something

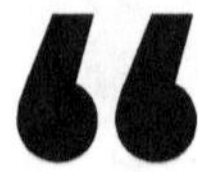

Do not confuse motion and progress.

- Alfred Montapert

"I'm just... I'm just not losing weight," Samantha said, dejected after her weight went up yet again.

"I'm eating better, moving more, drinking less... but it doesn't seem to make a difference. In fact, it's getting worse! I'm not sure what's going on."

As a health coach, it's a hard conversation to have when someone is paying you for a result and the opposite is happening. For whatever reason, we need to get to the root cause of why the body isn't responding as it should.

"Got it, Sam—you're frustrated. That's understandable when you're making changes but not seeing results. Let's dig into what's been happening. Last time we talked, you mentioned inconsistent meal planning, eating out a few times, and drinks with your boyfriend—sound about right?"

"Yeah, I guess I did. It was a rough week at work."

"You are under quite a deadline, that's for sure... I also saw a couple of missed workouts in our fitness app. Did you happen to get any of those in and forget to log it?"

"No, I missed them. Again, work took up long hours. I just couldn't get away from my desk as much as I would've liked... and besides that, I don't like my apartment complex's gym."

"We have been talking about finding a new gym for some time now... have you been taking work breaks to get sunshine and more steps in?"

"Well no... again, not as often as I'd like."

By now, we were both starting to see that the perception and the reality may not have been as tightly aligned as originally estimated.

"But I know I've been doing better!" Samantha said in a final attempt at reconciling her lack of progress.

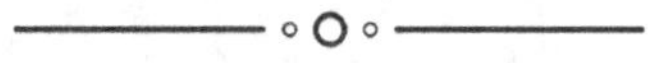

Writing down goals and fantasizing about a transformed future is easy—just ask the millions of people who do it every New Year ("champagne wishes," I call them). Goal execution and results are another story.

In order to get to a specific outcome, we've got to be related to the "what's so" on our journey.

Samantha's plight is not an unfamiliar one to me or probably you, dear reader.

Our personal bias leaves us nearly always thinking we've been living exclusively off salads, and conveniently forgetting the impact DoorDashing our favorite restaurant food a few times per week (at 9:00 pm) has on our waistline.

And hey, sometimes just generally doing "better" can work! That's what this book is about. If you don't exercise, starting to walk or lift weights will most likely yield a positive outcome. Trading an apple for chips or water for soda will yield a positive outcome.

But if we want to move the needle with precision and speed, we've got to get on the court, in the arena, by tracking our most important actions.

To lose weight: Create a nutrition plan and track how closely you follow it.

To get stronger or add more muscle: Create a training routine and add a little more weight to each exercise every week.

To get better sleep: Follow a routine and keep a journal on your nightstand to track your bed/wake times.

It doesn't have to be complicated, only consistent.

While there are myriad wellness and habit-tracking apps to utilize, a simple spreadsheet (digital or printed) with goals listed and a daily checkbox to mark progress can be a wonderful way to see whether the actions we take are moving us toward our desired outcomes.

Because data doesn't lie—and it's often the only way to really know where we stand on the journey toward those outcomes.

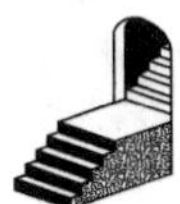

BOTTOM LINE:

- "The first principle is that you must not fool yourself—and you are the easiest person to fool."

- Cognitive bias leads us to believe we're doing more of the "good" stuff and less of the "bad" stuff, even if it's not accurate.

- Use one of the many habit tracking apps or devices (or plain old paper and pencil) to track how well you're actually doing. Until it's an ingrained habit, anything less than that is just hoping for the best.

Be mindful of what you put on your skin, hair, teeth and laundry

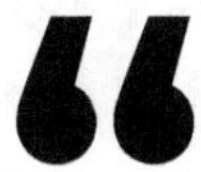

An ounce of prevention is worth a pound of cure.

- Benjamin Franklin

"Frank, what the hell is going on with your skin?"

I asked incredulously, walking into our dorm room and staring down a swath of angry red welts across his shirtless midsection. He was at his desk, rubbing his body and looking nervous.

"I don't know man... I just finished drying a load of laundry, threw on a clean t-shirt, and started studying... a few minutes later my whole body was itchy and puffy... kind of freaking out right now."

Judging by the smell of the freshly laundered clothes in our tiny dorm, I had a suspicion about the culprit.

"... Did you wash those clothes with a new kind of detergent?"

"Yeah, my mom just sent me a jug."

"Let me see it..."

It was a leading household brand, "fresh spring scent"... I could smell the noxious aroma without even opening the bottle.

Being raised by a Mom with hypersensitivity to detergents, fabric softeners, and synthetic fragrances had me on high alert for products like these.

"Dude, this stuff is poison." I pointed to the offending jug. "Shower up, get that off your skin, and re-wash your clothes with this instead," I said, handing him my hypoallergenic, fragrance-free option.

"Wait... What does that have to do with these welts?"

"Everything, dude. That detergent and 'spring fresh' scent is nothing but chemicals your body is having a reaction to."

"Okayyy, but it's supposed to be cleaning my clothes, right?"

"Yes, but the question is, what else is in there besides detergent?"

Sadly, the United States maintains some of the poorest standards in the western world when it comes to regulating the use of synthetic chemicals in consumer products.

That's right—much of what we clean our bodies and homes with leaves us at risk for skin irritations, headaches, brain fog, asthma, and even cancers.

By and large, behemoth, influential businesses have put profit over purpose, filling our shopping aisles with products that barrage our senses with fragrances and irritants.

Look no further than the fact that the European Union, Japan, and other countries have banned or limited more than 1,600 chemicals from personal care products, but regulators at the Food and Drug Administration prohibit just nine for safety reasons (at the time of this writing).[7] Yikes.

Here are just a few potentially harmful chemicals to watch out for:

Phthalates: Fixatives in fragranced products (deodorants, soaps, shampoos, lotions). EPA marks as "probable human carcinogens." Banned in Europe.

Triclosan: Antibacterial agent and registered pesticide. Disrupts thyroid and estrogen function.

BHA (Butylated Hydroxyanisole): Preservative in cosmetics and moisturizers. Endocrine disruptor. Banned in Europe.

Formaldehyde: Preservative found in shampoos, shower gels, baby wipes. "Known human carcinogen." Banned in Japan and Sweden.

Parabens: Preservatives in lotions, makeup, anti-aging products. Estrogen mimicking agent. Banned in Denmark for children's products.

When it comes to home and body care products, we've got to presume guilt before innocence.

The great news is consumers are beginning to demand healthier alternatives in shopping aisles, and more mainstream options are showing up. In many instances these "greener" products can be just as effective without the harmful side effects.

To ensure you're buying a healthier alternative, look for these certifications on the label:

- **Safer Choice** (EPA) — The Environmental Protection Agency's list of home cleaning products that meet their rigorous safety standards.

- **EcoLogo-certified** — Third party certification that indicates a product has undergone rigorous scientific testing and exhaustive auditing to prove its compliance with stringent environmental standards.

- **Green Seal certified** — Third party certification that verifies the product in hand uses safer chemicals, responsible sourcing, and other sustainability requirements.

- **EWG Verified** — Product is free from "ingredients of concern," fully discloses all ingredients, and meets stringent quality standards.

- **Made Safe** — Nonprofit certification that screens products for known and suspected toxicants harmful to humans and the environment.

- **B Corp** — Certifies the company meets high environmental, governance and cultural standards.

- **Certified Allergy & Asthma Friendly** — Tested and free of irritants and VOCs that could trigger asthma or allergies.

- **National Eczema Association (NEA) Seal of Acceptance** — Tested and certified to be free of dyes, fragrances, and certain preservatives known to cause skin sensitivity.

Or simply make your own! A combination of vinegar, baking soda, lemon, and essential oils can take care of many house cleaning needs. Castile soap, glycerin, and essential oils create a simple body wash. Simply do a search for "natural cleaner/body wash recipes," and you'll find many to choose from.

If homesteading isn't your thing, visit EWG.org, a consumer health watchdog group, to see how home and beauty products rate based on the safety of their ingredients, as well as safer alternative options to consider.

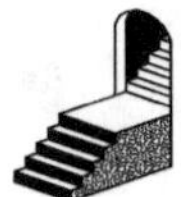

BOTTOM LINE:

- Transitioning to cleaner home and personal products has never been easier. They're usually not much more expensive than conventional options, and the upcharge is well worth the upside.

- Look for labels with certifications on their packaging to denote quality assurance.

- Use EWG.org as a launch point to determine if a particular product is worthy of a place on your body and in your home.

Plan your meals and snacks

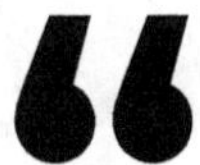

A goal without a plan is just a wish.

- Antoine de Saint-Exupéry

"I'm doing this... am I really doing this?

You just said it was on your goals list. What the hell are you waiting for?"

Enters credit card. Click. Click. Paid.

"I'm really doing this."

I had just entered my first physique show at the behest of Alan, my designated accountability partner during a coaching program.

Alan was a no nonsense Jewish guy from the east coast—straight shooter to the core.

At this point, our program had us taking on a big, juicy challenge or goal to accomplish in three months or less. Competing in a physique show was something I had entertained, but was admittedly intimidated by.

I had a nice body at the time, but was it show-worthy? That's what made me hesitate.

"Okay... registered—what do I do now?"

"I dunno man, but you've got about 11 weeks to find out," Alan said with a wry smile.

A week later, I'd hired Sean, a natural bodybuilder in my network who had won multiple competitions, as my coach.

"Lifting weights will be crucial to maintain your physique, but the gains will be negligible at this point before the show. The key will be to master your food intake and get you as lean as possible," Sean said. "Here's your food plan, grocery list, and meal times when I want you to eat. Stick with this, and you'll have a shot to compete on stage."

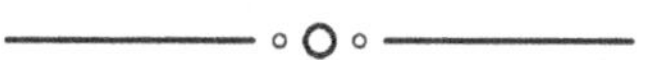

I knew I had to get a tight handle on my food game when I started doing physique shows. There was just no way to trust what I was eating without cooking it myself when I needed to have 4% body fat so quickly.

Restaurant and prepared foods are not only expensive, they are also often fraught with cheap inflammatory oils, too much sodium, and too many hidden calories. And this isn't even mentioning the oft-huge portion sizes!

I wasn't going there.

To lean out for my show, I would eat the same thing every day: eggs and oatmeal for breakfast; lean ground turkey or chicken breast with mustard, rice with garlic salt, and broccoli (or another green) for lunch and dinner. Before bed, I'd have more oatmeal and whey protein to put on weight between shows. Seven days per week.

It was an effective way to lose body fat. I got down to 4% body fat and placed fourth in my first show!

I did two more shows within the year, doing nearly the same food plan almost every day.

While I really liked having a lean body that came with the practice of mindful food preparation, eating that plainly and routinely became painfully boring—so much so I stopped competing because food consumption became all-consuming.

After a period of indulgence and self-sabotage (I needed pizza and beer, dammit!), I finally found the sweet spot that keeps 80-85% of the results with 25% of the effort.

It's the best way I've found that allows some dietary flexibility while still maintaining the tenets of eating heartily and healthily for most meals of the week, with a reprieve on the weekends.

Here's our weekly plan:

Write out a menu for the week. One protein, one starch, one or two vegetables per meal, five meals in total if you like to have more freedom on the weekends. If you're stuck on meal inspiration, Whole30, Paleo, and Primal Kitchen are great places to find healthy options. You can also do a Google search for recipes to prepare meals with, making the search healthier by adding "+ Paleo" at the end of the description to find less processed options. Lately, we've been using ChatGPT to make our meal plan and the attendant grocery list—it makes the process a breeze. Double the recipe amounts so you've got lunch for the next day. Be sure to include snacks such as fruit, veggie sticks, meal replacement/protein bars (we like TruBars, IQ Bars and LaraBars), string cheese, mixed nuts, oatmeal, low sugar yogurt, hummus, and guacamole packets. We stick to the perimeter of the grocery store for almost everything—the middle is where most of the junk is. We buy organic when able.

Shop for the main ingredients. Wholesalers like Costco and Sam's Club are a family's blessing if you have one in your area. Then, swing by a standard grocer for the few specialty items you can't get in bulk. I suggest taking a couple of hours out on a Saturday or Sunday and make it an event to look forward to. Bring your partner or family along to be part of the process—they'll appreciate having input!

Cook it and eat it: Sounds obvious, but this is where people get stuck. It's like buying a gym membership and never going—except your fridge full of groceries costs way more.

The key? Actually cook the food.

Some people batch-cook on Sundays, freeze meals, and pull one out daily. But most people just cook one day at a time—and that's fine. Crockpots are your friend here. Throw ingredients in before work, set to low, come home to dinner ready.

Have the family help or be part of the process. Chopping, peeling, cleaning, all goes more quickly and smoothly in partnership. Or you can alternate cooking days if you've got a willing partner.

Food management can be the most time-intensive practice in this book, and unquestionably the most important.

However, our family food prep practice doesn't always make sense if you just cook for one or two people (or don't like grocery shopping, etc.).

For those readers, here are a few hacks to employ:

Grocery delivery: If you don't want to take the time to shop, many grocers now offer low cost delivery service or free pickup. Simply go to their website, pick out the items on your list, and arrange to have them picked up/dropped off at a scheduled time. You can often save lists if you tend to order similar things week in and week out. While there are drawbacks (you may be stuck with imperfect produce, occasional wrong items, or substitutions), this one saves time if it's the shopping and commute that are holding you back.

Meal delivery service: This is the way to go if you've got a little extra coin or are just cooking for one. You can have all or some of your meals made and dropped off at your door. Simply select a plan based on goals, choose from the company's weekly rotating menu of options and you're done. Cost typically ranges $10-14 per meal. Simply type "meal delivery service + your city" to get started. Many offer discounted plans to first time subscribers, so try out a few and see which one you like best.

Pre-made proteins: Proteins typically take the longest to cook and prepare. Some companies now offer protein-only subscription services. For just a few dollars per serving, you can have canned, pre-marinated proteins delivered and ready to eat. Many grocers have pre-made proteins in the frozen aisle (just be on the lookout for hidden sugars and suspect ingredients here!). Other ready-to-eat proteins I like are sardines and mackerel (in olive oil), line-caught tuna (lower mercury), and the occasional rotisserie chicken. I know none of these are perfect options, but conviction and convenience don't live on the same block, ya dig?

Whatever your version of food planning, aim to include these essentials (portions are per person):

- (1-2) 4-ounce/palmful-sized portions of protein at lunch and dinner

- (1-2) cups/fist-sized portions of vegetables at every meal

- (1-2) ½ cup/cupped palm portions of a starch at lunch and a little less at dinner if you want to lose fat

- (1-2) tablespoons/thumb-sized portions of fat

For snacks: Majority whole food (fruits, veggie sticks, yogurt and cheese, nuts, and raisins in moderation).

The key is to have them close by and at the ready! Eating healthily is so much easier when the environment is conducive to do so.

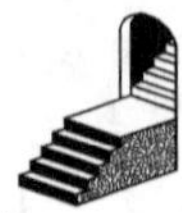

BOTTOM LINE:

- Whether you do it all at once or on a daily basis, cooking can and will take a few hours, but there is nothing more important to long-term health than the quality and quantity of food we eat.

- Don't rely on Uber Eats or restaurants to attain the health and body you want.

- There are ways to save time without sacrificing quality. Find your system and stick with it.

- Visit **www.eattheapplebook.com** for a free video tutorial on how to use ChatGPT as a grocery shopping and recipe-generating assistant.

Prep your life
the night before

Failing to prepare is preparing to fail.

- John Wooden

Mike texted me minutes before our session was set to begin.

So sorry, Derek. I need to cancel again. I've got a mountain of discovery to read, multiple HR trainings to complete,and I haven't even begun to prepare for my deposition tomorrow morning! Going to be another late one :(Hope to see you next week...

He had hit a tipping point. The firm he worked for was bought by a much larger one. He lost a few of his best partners who had previously shared the workload. He was getting married. He was missing work-outs and eating late-night comfort food. Stress was mounting.

Life was moving faster than he could keep up with.

A few weeks passed like this, with Mike either missing sessions or showing up tardy and discombobulated. Until one day he showed up to our session early.

"Mike, you're here—on time!"

"Can you believe it!?" he said with a laugh.

"I'm thrilled—what changed?"

"With all of the craziness going on, I had to take a serious look at how I was using my time—especially in the evenings. I was so exhausted and drained after work, I'd just flop on the couch and watch TV until midnight. The longer night would have me wake up later with nothing prepared, leaving me racing to catch up with my to-do list. It's been unsustainable. So I started preparing for the next morning right after work was done to make sure I had my well-being handled. I also set an alarm to get me away from the TV and into bed by 9:30."

"Wow!" I said. "How do you feel?"

"Yeah! I feel revitalized. While the workload and wedding planning are still intense, I'm glad to have some healthy habits on autopilot that help me handle it all."

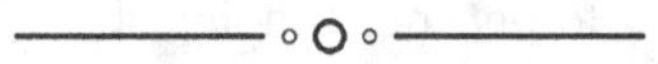

When it comes to performing at a high level day in and day out, the healthiest of us consistently execute their plan for their next day's success. Much of the routine practices are simple—banal, even. Of the dozens of steps suggested in this book so far, many of them can be condensed and put into a structure with roughly 20-30 minutes of preparatory time before bed.

Make your smoothie: ten minutes. Prepare your lunch and snacks for the next day: seven minutes. Refill your water bottle: one minute. Take out your outfit the night before: one minute. Walk a little after dinner or stretch before bed: ten minutes. Pack your gym clothes for the next day: one minute. Quick to-do list for the next day: two minutes.

Simple as these steps are, it never ceases to amaze me how often nobody does them!

Yet, executing a few simple practices and preparations the night before is what makes all the difference in attaining and maintaining a healthy lifestyle with ease.

People who say they don't have time to be healthy often can't tell you what they do with their evenings.

"Oh, well, I don't know. I usually put the kids down then watch some television or scroll on my phone and then go to bed. I'm usually too tired to do much of anything else after work and kids."

Yet, the healthy habit they are not doing is the very same thing that will bring them more energy and focus without wasted effort!

Routines remove the superfluous thinking about what to eat, how much water to drink, or whether one has brought a change of clothes to exercise in.

Make your next day easier with a little forethought the evening prior— the planning pays for itself many times over. I promise having a routine down pat will provide a lot more satisfaction than watching another TV show.

No matter your schedule, an evening routine makes it way easier to stick with the healthy habits that tend to fall off the radar—sleep prep, meal planning, movement, wind-down time.

Ever go on a work trip, forget your running shoes, and then can't go to the gym or on a run?

How about being stuck at the airport with nothing but unhealthy options to eat before your flight?

Ever stand in front of your pantry working from home, finding yourself grazing on all your kids' snacks?

We're more likely to miss or skip steps during a rushed morning of meetings or getting kids out the door than when we take a few minutes the night before to make sure what we need to handle gets handled.

Having a container of what I'm going to eat, drink, and wear to the gym and work helps me avoid snacking on junk food, helps me drink more water so I'm fully hydrated, and signals to my brain that I'm going to get my butt to the gym after work is done.

Seek out anyone who has a busy life and a physique you admire. I'll bet they will tell you they've got a rock-solid evening routine that keeps their health humming without too much thought.

Like Will Durant (paraphrasing Aristotle) wrote: "We are what we repeatedly do... therefore excellence is not an act, but a habit."

Here are my evening to-do's (after dinner and cleaning up the kitchen):

- Pack whatever was for dinner that evening for lunch the next day. Protein, starch, fat, veggies.

- Prep snacks (an apple and orange, raw mixed nuts, a quality protein bar, or homemade muffin).

- Prep breakfast (overnight oats and smoothies—I'll typically prep multiple days at a time to only do it every other day or so).

- Fill up two 24-oz water bottles and add electrolyte or mineral blend to one.

- Prep supplements. Fish oil, vegetable powder blend, creatine, amino acids.

- Gym clothes, fresh socks, and training sneakers.

- Write down anything positive worth remembering from the day and drop a note into my jar of awesome.

- Quick brain dump on a to-do list for the next day to clear my mind before sleep.

- Thank God for the abundance bestowed upon me and my family.

That's it!

Sometimes I'll go for a walk after dinner or a stretch in the living room if the kids are calm, but Sunday through Thursday that's my routine.

Food, hydration, fitness, and mindfulness all accounted for in the time it takes to watch a sitcom.

And *voila!* We await the next day prepared and empowered.

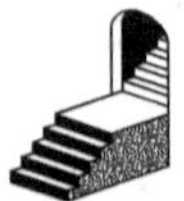

BOTTOM LINE:

- The body and health you want are on the other side of executing your evening routine.

- Don't let your mornings go off the rails. Fool-proof your unpredictable mornings by laying out everything you need for a healthy day the night before.

- Have a look at your schedule—make sure you've got steps in place to manage food, hydration, fitness, and mindfulness before bedtime.

- Visit **www.eattheapplebook.com** for a free downloadable "Excellent Evening" checklist.

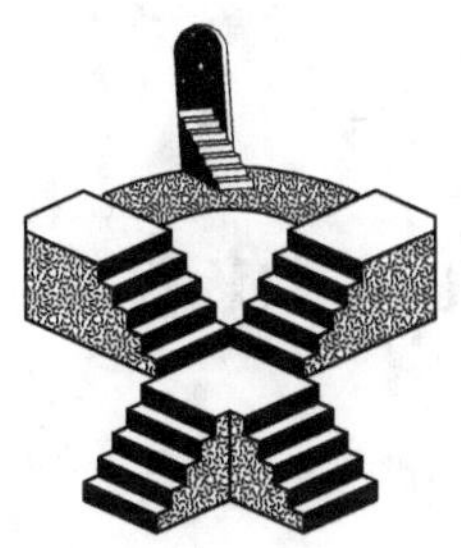

FIFTH FLIGHT

Fast, but not too much

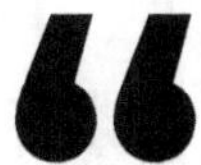

> # Fasting is the greatest remedy - the physician within.
>
> - Paracelsus

"Now remember, Olga, it's important that you eat 6 small meals per day. This helps maintain blood sugar levels. So be sure to eat every 2-3 hours, okay?"

Olga was my first personal training client after getting my first certification (poor thing). She was a kind, heavy-set Russian woman who just wanted to lose 30 lbs before going on a cruise with her girlfriends. Simple enough, right?

Alas, the road to hell is paved with good intentions...

In a thick, Russian accent, she said, doubtfully, "Derek, I don't know. It seems like a lot of food."

She wasn't wrong. Eating to that extent (especially cleanly) is a lot of work and a lot of food.

"Trust me, Olga. This is the best way to do it," I said with blind confidence.

Well, three months and a hundred meals too many later, she hadn't lost a pound.

We were both sad, confused.

She hadn't lost weight; I had lost a client.

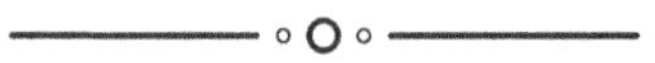

Fasting: Adverb. Definition: "To abstain from all kinds of food or drink."

Fasting has gotten a lot of attention in the media lately—some good, some curious, some bad.

Many media stories (with a negative bent against fasting) point to fasting (intermittent or extended) as being a detriment toward health due to:

- Elevated strain on the heart and cardiovascular systems

- Nausea, headaches, lightheadedness

- Extreme hunger

In some ways the stories are correct. Too much fasting in the wrong environment, under extreme circumstances is bad for your health.

When done incorrectly, fasting causes cortisol (your stress hormone) to spike. Add in common mistakes—exercising too much, eating too little during feeding windows, or bingeing on unhealthy food—and the whole thing backfires. People end up with hunger/overeating cycles, low energy, and brain fog. Eventually, they quit and write fasting off as "too hard" or "not for me."

I've seen this play out too many times to count.

However, with the right structure and planning, fasting can be a simple, regenerative practice, allowing us to intentionally slow down, rejuvenate, and even heal ourselves.

Just like anything and everything, the devil is in the details. Let me break down the two main types of fasting and what each is good for:

Intermittent Fasting

What is it:

- Fasting for 12-18 hours. I recommend staying closer to 12-14 hours—16-18 is too aggressive for most people, despite being popular.

What is it good for:

- **Calorie/food intake management:** Great for habitual snackers and anxious eaters.

- **Blood sugar regulation**

- **Sleep quality:** Allowing space between eating and bedtime is crucial for sleep quality. Eating right before bed (or even 2 hours or less if consuming a large meal) can greatly impact sleep. The digestive process requires energy—approximately 10-15% of total daily calories through what's called the thermic effect of food—meaning our organs can't fully rest if they're still working to process recently eaten food.[1]

Extended Fasting

What is it:

- 24 hours or more of food abstinence

What is it good for:

- **Quelling inflammation:** Inflammatory biomarkers such as high blood sugar, hemoglobin A1c, C-reactive protein, Lipopolysaccharide levels, and many more can be reduced by entering a fasted state.

- **Healing digestion:** It is said that approximately six out of 10 people experience some sort of digestive issue on a regular or semi-regular basis[2]. Digestive issues can stem from a myriad of conditions or environments: inflammatory foods that don't agree with our bodies, chronic stress, over-exercising, and non-steroidal anti-inflammatory drugs like Advil, birth control, or even chronic systemic issues, such as Hashimoto's. By refraining from eating, we remove the inputs that are exacerbating our digestive discomfort, and allow our digestive lining to heal the lamina propria of our small intestine, where the majority of our digestion and often digestive issues occur. (The lamina propria, which separates our small intestine from our blood stream, is only two cells thick and thus vulnerable to digestive disruptions.)

- **Autophagy:** Meaning "self-eating" in Greek, is the body's process designed to remove dead or dying cells (cellular senescence) and recycle the usable components of damaged cells.

- **Activating Adenosine Monophosphate Protein Kinase (AMPK) pathways:** Which supports fatty acid and glucose metabolism.

- **Detoxification:** Fasting for extended periods supports the liver and kidneys to cleanse and purify the toxins that are already circulating in our system, allowing those detoxification organs to not have to focus on incoming food and drink. The liver is responsible for over 500 processes within the body, many of them related to detoxification. When we don't eat or drink (or eat and drink very little) it allows our liver (and to a lesser extent kidneys) the time to focus on cleaning out what is already inside our bodies.

As you can see, there are a lot of benefits to implementing a regular fasting practice.

However, we've got to make sure we're set up for success in order to make fasting a regular part of our health routine—otherwise we'll become hungry, stressed out, or experience symptoms like dizziness and low blood sugar.

Here are a few tips I've found remarkably supportive for myself and my clients to make implementing a fasting practice more approachable and effective.

Intermittent Fasting Tips

Start with a 12 hour fast: Stop eating two hours before bed, sleep eight hours, don't eat or drink anything with calories for two hours after waking up, and *voila!* You've got yourself a 12 hour fast. Once you've implemented that, consider increasing it up to two more hours (up to 14 hours—more effective if fat loss is your goal).

Hydrate with mineral rich, purified water, especially in the morning: As mentioned, fasting is excellent for detoxification. Hydration is also a crucial component of detoxification. Ensuring you start your day with a large glass or bottle of water helps further dispose of the toxins we accumulate as we rest.

Add a lemon wedge for a boost of potassium and to wake up your digestive tract in anticipation of food to come. This point is crucial for those with weak digestion—i.e., those who don't do well digesting red meats and cruciferous vegetables (such as broccoli, cabbage, and Brussels sprouts)—as lemon water helps build the gastric juices of the stomach. If you identify as a high stress person, throw in a pinch of quality salt, such as Redmond, Colima or Celtic salt to replace minerals used by the adrenal system.

You can also add in a zero calorie mineral additive such as Trace Minerals or Jigsaw's adrenal cocktail, which are high in potassium, magnesium, and quality sodium.

If you're a coffee fanatic, drink water and wait at least an hour after waking to have your first cup: Caffeine stimulates our central nervous system, which can re-elevate cortisol. I know, it pains me to wait too, but the benefits are vast. Plus, the coffee hits better when consumed a little later.

For the Ladies: The best time to start a fasting practice is during or right after your period, when hormone levels are at their lowest. Women have much more to consider than men in this realm, so it's important to be mindful about timing.

Extended Fasting Tips

All of the above apply, AND:

Plan for it: Choose a day, weekend, or day of the week that you know will have very few plans. Don't plan on doing much but resting. If you have young children, do your best to plan for low-key days with movies, board games, crafts, and easy walks in the neighborhood. In fact, these are good activities to plan for with or without children.

Start with a 24 hour fast: I like doing the dinner time to dinner time fasting protocol. One gets good benefits from the prolonged abstinence, but dinner time is not so far away as to have you chew your hand off in hunger or anxiety.

Replenish your vitamins, minerals, and amino acids during your fasting window: Most people miss this. Keeping your micronutrients and amino acids topped off helps you handle stress, protect muscle mass, and gives you a little flavor to make fasting less boring. I add 1-2 servings of amino acids daily—they're key for preserving muscle. (I use Kion, but any quality amino acid supplement works.)

You can even eat a little of the right foods(!): That's right—research has shown one can follow a 5-day, low-calorie protocol and still yield vast benefits of fasting without going sans food completely. Research by Valter Longo, director of the University of Southern California's Longevity Institute, demonstrates we can yield nearly all of the benefits of fasting while still keeping our sanity through the process.[3]

I like a scoop of EquiLife's Daily Nutritional Support powder mixed with 12 to 16 ounces of water four times throughout the fast. This provides me with the vitamins and minerals needed, some protein to spare muscle wasting, and stimulates my tastebuds throughout the day.

To experience even greater benefits: You can extend the fasting window to 48-72 hours by repeating the 24-hour protocol—just skip dinner each day and continue with the supplements and hydration.

With the right planning, it's really not that challenging! Plus, the long-term benefits are among the most powerful health practices available. Try one to two extended fasts per year on calm weekends. You'll be so glad you did.

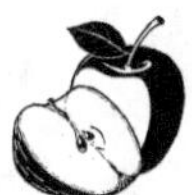

BOTTOM LINE:

- Fasting when done properly, can be the closest thing to a fountain of youth we've got.

- Start with a 12 hour fast, spacing the time more so after dinner to improve sleep quality if possible.

- Ladies, pay heed to your cycle timing when advancing intermittent or extended fasting protocols.

- Hydrate with purified, mineral rich water and wait to drink coffee.

- Plan your extended fasts during times with as little to do as possible, communicating your intentions with friends and family.

- Start small and grow practice until finding your sweet spot.

Do an "S" per day

> **Remember, daily exercise is a must. Plan for it, and do it. The rewards will be well worth it.**
>
> - Jack LaLanne

"I love to run, man. I run four miles every day before work. It's my happy place and sets my day up for success," Mira told me during our wellness consultation.

"I've been doing it for years and want to keep it as part of my routine. I reached out to you because I'd like to get stronger and have more muscle. The trouble is I don't know what I'm doing in the weight room. I don't know where to begin, how much to lift... frankly I'm a little nervous about injuring myself. So I just stick to my run five days per week and avoid that part of the gym altogether."

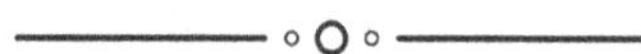

It can be so hard to know where to begin when going through an exercise program.

"Well, I want to lose weight, but my lower back hurts..."

"I do like to run, but it's been a long time since I've done that..."

"Maybe I should strength train first? But I don't even know what I'm doing!"

For many, the thought of going to a gym or beginning an exercise plan can feel daunting, especially if one doesn't have much experience or confidence to begin with.

With all of the information available on where to begin, it can feel overwhelming—scary, even.

For simplicity's sake, I recommend that all my new clients start with an **S per day**—one of the following: **stretch, sweat, or strength.**

A well-rounded physique can perform in all three realms. Each modality has wonderful aspects about it, yet none is fully complete.

In my opinion, mobility practices like yoga don't stimulate enough muscle growth or challenge the aerobic system.

Aerobic work is wonderful for heart health and mental health, but does very little for your mobility or muscular development, especially in the upper body.

Strength training is key for muscular development and bone density, but does less for heart health and total body mobility (especially for beginners).

All are excellent... and incomplete.

Enter: the S per day.

Here's how to build a simple movement plan:

Monday—Stretch: Yoga class or 25-minute YouTube video.
S #1: Check.

Tuesday—Sweat: Brisk walk, run, jump rope—anything that gets your heart rate up. **S #2: Check.**

Wednesday—Strength: Gym, home bodyweight workout, resistance bands—doesn't matter. Just challenge your muscles. **S #3: Check.**

Once you've hit all three, loop back to Monday. (Or take a rest day and restart.)

This isn't perfect, but it's simple and covers everything. Eventually you'll combine S's into single workouts. For now? Your body cares way more about consistency than perfection.

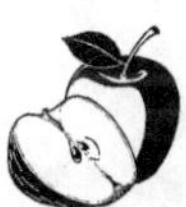

BOTTOM LINE:

- It's important to sweat, stretch, and strengthen. Each focus brings a distinct, crucial aspect of health the others are missing.

- Health is a long game. Give yourself the time and space to do a different kind of movement each day, and you'll be much more prone to sticking with the plan versus burning yourself out performing just one (incomplete) modality.

- Visit **eattheapplebook.com** to download your "Daily S" workout guide.

Maximize your commute

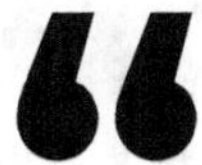

> # The key is not in spending time, but investing it.
>
> - Stephen Covey

"Do we really have to move? Our life is set up here... I know it will be a little cramped, but I think we can do it!" I pleaded with my wife, meekly and sheepishly.

"Derek, we're having another child. We can't stay in this tiny home any longer."

Deep down I knew she was right. We had lived in our cute but oh-so-small two-bedroom, one-bathroom home for the last five years. While it was manageable with three of us, packing in a baby and everything that comes with a baby was clearly stressing out my wife.

After long deliberation and consideration, the opportunity arose to move to a beautiful, four-bedroom three-bathroom home. It was perfect. The only problem... it was 42 miles away from my work.

When Joslyn proposed this idea to me I got a lump in my throat. "A 42-mile commute? Each way? That's insane."

I was heavily resisting this fact, and starting to dig my heels in. Maybe the kids could get bunk beds after all?

"I know that's a lot for you and you'll be making the biggest sacrifice out of all of us to make this change. But I just don't see how we can make it work in our neighborhood with the expense of moving into a bigger house."

She was right again. We had moved into an area that had become exponentially more expensive than when we had arrived, and suddenly found ourselves priced out of our own neighborhood.

With a big sigh and a load of resistance still to carry, I relented and we moved into our beautiful home... 42 miles from my work.

I was initially riled about the commute, to no one's surprise. Car time had effectively more than doubled, so I spent the first few weeks just resenting my wife and my kids for pulling me further away. Don't for a second think I wrote this chapter without struggle.

When I finally calmed down, I considered what my commute was previously—listening to the news, mindless podcasts, biting my nails, spacing out.

A lot of wasted time, to be honest.

Next, I thought—'What could it look like to develop myself while going through the commute?'

Here's what I came up with:

- Learn more about my profession—I could obtain continuing education credits. Learners are earners.

- Pleasure reading—With a young family and career, my time to read had dwindled. This is my chance to make up some ground with audiobooks.

- Develop better hair, skin, and nails—I bite my nails most when I'm driving. I've got to beat that habit... and I can surely work on these 40-year-old crow's feet and hairline.

- Connect with out-of-state family and friends—Life has certainly made it harder to call family in a quiet setting. My parents aren't getting any younger...

- Breathwork—This was once part of my morning routine... I really liked doing it. What happened?

- Get curious about driving posture—Unconscious driving throws my hip and neck out of whack...

"Come to think of it, there might be some ways to actually make this commute useful after all!"

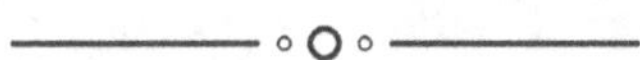

America is a driving country. The average commute? 55 minutes per day, roundtrip.[4] Nearly 10 days a year sitting in your car. And that's not counting the stress—traffic jams, construction zones, aggressive drivers. All of it spiking cortisol.

However, unless we can convince our boss to let us work remotely or change jobs that move us closer to home, commuting will remain a staple of our lives.

But hey—if you can't beat 'em, join 'em. There's always an opportunity to optimize!

Here are my drive time routines:

To work:

- 1 minute: Before starting the engine, apply anti-biting nail polish and face cream

- 5 minutes: Breathwork (eyes open, obviously!)—I transition between box breathing (4 counts inhale - 4 counts hold - 4 counts exhale - 4 counts hold) and breath of fire (2 quick inhales, one exhale)

- 10 minutes: Red light therapy cap for hair growth

- 15 minutes: Inspirational podcast—Something to get in the right mindset.

- 15-20 minutes: Training and development via podcast or health/coaching continuing education.

Back home:

- Hydrate: Catch up on any water deficit if my bottle is still full

- Snack: Anything left in my lunchbox

- Phone call or two to friends or family

- Rub my "massage" stone: A flat blue calcite (known for calming) to help prevent nail picking and biting. Re-apply polish and moisturize hands.

- Small dose of news consumption.

And making a point throughout the drive to notice:

- **Posture:** Feet up, hips square, sitting tall through spine, shoulders dropped.

- **Breathing** (perpetually, not just doing breath work): Inhaling and exhaling through the nose, into the belly with relaxed jaw and face.

- **Thoughts:** Am I at peace? If I'm not, can I choose it in the midst of this traffic?

After a few weeks the habits began to set in. I was happy to find more purpose and function in the drive. The dedicated structure in place for my commutes transformed my productivity and relationship to the time I'm in the car.

Don't get me wrong, a 90 minute commute home on a Friday afternoon still sucks sometimes. I occasionally struggle to maintain a positive, resilient attitude upon arriving home for my family. Regardless of my "feelings" on a given day, the opportunities are there to improve myself physically and mentally with better use of time available.

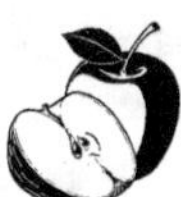

BOTTOM LINE:

■ Most Americans—87%—commute to work.[5] Most of them drive. That's time in the car. Every single day. What you do with it matters.

Look at your poops

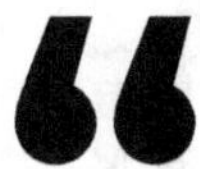

Happiness: a good bank account, a good cook, and a good digestion.

- Jean-Jacques Rousseau

"Truth be told, I've had intermittent constipation and diarrhea most of my life... not sure what causes either. It just kind of... happens."

Carol confided in me on one of our first coaching sessions. I asked her to expound more on the subject after her intake form indicated some bowel movement irregularities.

"I think I eat well—at least during the week. Restaurants are kind of my weekend thing... but lo and behold, my digestion is all over the place."

"Ok, got that—you've had a hard time pinning down what's causing the irregularities. Have you ever thought to track your bowel movements?"

"Huh? Ummm no."

"Weird question, I realize, and believe it or not, what our poop looks like communicates a lot about our health at large."

"Really? I try not to think about it too much."

"You and nearly everybody else! I'm aware of the strange request, but simply by making two or three lifestyle adjustments, most clients find they start to yield a better-formed, more consistent and easy-to-pass stool in just a few short weeks—sometimes even sooner. And when that's back on track, you'll really begin to notice a difference in diges-tive comfort, bloating, and overall life satisfaction. With that in mind, would you be open to tracking your poops so we can start to see what may be causing the inconsistencies?"

Pauses

"My boyfriend will be thrilled to finally have an excuse to talk about poop at the dinner table. I didn't expect this request, but yes, yes let's do it."

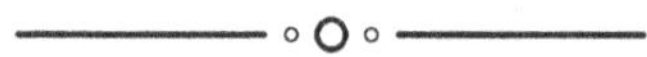

Taboo as the scatological topic can be, poop is one of the most effective and immediate biomarkers we can use to assess our health.

There are a lot of moving parts that go into digesting the food we eat. Many things can go awry along the tract with so many factors at play.

Yet stool form and color can:

- Hold clues toward discovering one's root cause of bowel dysfunction (if there is some irregularity)

- Potentially improve the quality and consistency

- Help you know when to go to a doctor

Here's a breakdown of what some of the more common poop textures and colors can say about your health, according to the Bristol Stool Chart, a visual reference guide:

Type 1: Pebbles. **Appearance:** Hard and separate little lumps that look like nuts and are hard to pass. **Indicates:** These little pellets typically mean you're constipated. It shouldn't happen frequently. Dehydration, lack of movement, eating too much animal protein, not enough fiber or slowed motility due to stress may all be factors here.

Type 2: Caterpillar **Appearance:** Log-shaped but hard lumpy; perhaps requiring increased effort to pass. **Indicates:** A sign of constipation that, again, shouldn't happen frequently. Lack of hydration, not enough movement, too much animal protein vs. too few plants/fiber can be culprits to address.

Type 3: Sausage **Appearance:** Log-shaped with some cracks on the surface. **Indicates:** The gold standard of poop, especially if it's somewhat soft and easy to pass.

Type 4: Snake **Appearance:** Smooth and snake-like. **Indicates:** Healthy digestive function—doctors also consider this a quality, normal poop.

Type 5: Amoebas **Appearance:** Small, individual stool balls that are soft and easy to pass (maybe they evacuate quickly); the blobs also have clear-cut edges. **Could Indicate:** Lack of fiber, exercising too closely or intensely in proximity to eating.

Type 6: Frozen yogurt **Appearance:** Fluffy and mushy with undefined edges. **Could indicate:** A sign of mild diarrhea. Lack of fiber, lack of electrolytes, and reaction to spicy foods or intolerances to dairy, wheat, eggs, or a particular FODMAP food..

Type 7: Messy **Appearance:** Completely watery with no solid pieces. **Could indicate:** Surprise—you've got diarrhea. Your stool moved through your bowels too quickly and didn't form into a healthy poop. Rapid transit through the digestive tract can also mean reduced nutrient absorption, heightened stress response, too intense an exercise session, or intolerance to a specific food or ingredient.

Who knew poop form could say so much?! But there's more—stool color also communicates something about the state of digestion.

Brown: The color we ideally see, stemming from an appropriate combination of bile and bilirubin.

Yellow: Can also be due to eating high amounts of turmeric or beta-carotene-rich foods like sweet potatoes or squash. Potential trouble digesting fat due to liver issues or insufficient bile secretion from the gallbladder. Long-term yellow coloration could point to malabsorption issues such as celiac disease or lactose intolerance.

Black: You ate a dark-colored food (such as blueberries, beets, or black licorice), consumed an iron or charcoal supplement, or took a bismuth supplement. In some cases, it can also signal potential bleeding in the upper digestive tract—especially when accompanied by a tar-like texture, foul smell, or uncomfortable symptoms.

Green: You ate green foods containing chlorophyll, matcha, or the food is passing too fast and bile isn't in the tract for long enough to turn the stool brown. It could mean malabsorption is present.

Red: You ate red food (beets in particular). Bright red stool could indicate hemorrhoids or bleeding in the lower digestive tract.

Pale, clay-colored or white: You consumed certain medications like antacids or barium used during an X-ray, which can lead to temporary whitening. A bile duct may be blocked, or more serious liver conditions such as cirrhosis or hepatitis may also be at play.

Yet another set of clues!

Refer to the Bristol chart again—a brown three or four on this scale that's easy to push out is the color, consistency, and shape we strive for. If this is your typical poop one to three times daily, there's a good chance your digestive tract is functioning properly.

Don't panic if you see something different occasionally. Miscolored stool, temporary loose stool, or constipation can happen to almost everyone due to a variety of factors.

Let's start with some possible culprits:

Food choices:

- Fried or spicy foods can irritate the digestive tract and lead to diarrhea.

- Processed foods—highly manufactured, pesticide-laden, or synthetic ingredients can be hard for the body to effectively digest and lead to diarrhea.

- Not enough fiber—Insoluble fiber gives form and bulk to stool, slowing down food's movement through stomach and intestine. Soluble fiber absorbs excess water in the intestine, thus helping to prevent loose stool. Lack of either can typically lead to constipation.

- Too much fat—Bile breaks down fat in the digestive process. Increased fat consumption typically increases bile production. Too much bile dropped can irritate intestinal lining.

Food intolerance: Can be due to enzyme deficiencies (like lactase, the enzyme which breaks down milk's lactose) or irritation from food additives, causing diarrhea.

Dehydration: Leads to less water in the colon and slowed motility, causing the body to reabsorb water from the stool, which leads to hard-to-pass poops.

Stress: The gut-brain axis releases stress hormones (like adrenaline and cortisol) during "fight or flight," causing digestion to speed up (diarrhea) or slow down (constipation).

Not enough movement: Inactivity leads to longer stool transit time due to reduced digestive muscle stimulation, and thus increased chance of constipation.

Too much movement: Intense or prolonged exercise can redirect blood to the limbs (known as intestinal ischemia), as well as jostle organs to stimulate unexpected and immediate diarrhea.

As you can see, bowel movements bring a lot of factors into play.

Doctors say a day or two of irregularity isn't much to worry about. But longer-term, (lasting more than a few days to a week), changes in color and/or form should warrant further medical attention.

Regardless of your variety, stool form and color are valuable (and free) biomarkers to observe how one's health is currently faring. Take heed of what's in the bowl!

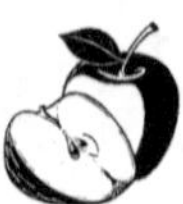

BOTTOM LINE:

- Bathroom visits can provide valuable insights into what your bowels say about your health in the short and long term.

- Note the Bristol Stool Chart and attendant "color matching" guide—3/4's and brown is the standard. Pay attention if anything else is showing up on a regular basis.

- Visit **www.eattheapplebook.com** for a downloadable Bristol Stool chart pdf.

Put your ass on the line: get in partnership

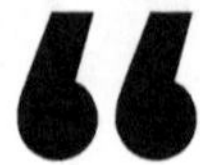

> # I get by with a little
> # help from my friends.
>
> – The Beatles

"Andreas- I've been stuck with this awful habit for almost 30 years; I'm really frustrated with myself. Like... why can't I get this under control?'

I'm a recovering nail and cuticle biter.

It would typically start with a worrisome thought, a serious conversation, or a moment where I need to take on a challenging mental task.

A deep, anxious, or out-of-control thought would have me focus on something I could simultaneously control and check out with—nail biting.

Trolling my finger tips, I'd pounce with a nibble or pick to remove an errant piece of cuticle skin or jagged nail edge. Once I did, I'd need to pick a little more to smooth out what I had already picked at, which would continue to expand the bitten area.

By the time I was through, my fingertip was a chewed, raw mess. Sometimes it bled.

I have tried so many times to quit.

Finger polish. Keeping hands moisturized. Wearing gloves while driving. Will power.

Nothing stuck.

Exasperated, in a vulnerable moment, I told a new friend, Andreas, about my plight. Until then I didn't know he was in Alcoholics Anonymous—over 20 years sober.

"Well, perhaps you could give yourself and the addiction up to God and get some support," he said to me.

"Huh?"

"There's a tenet in AA in which each person has a 'sponsor'—someone who has been through what you're going through—who helps support through the tough times. Sponsors are an integral part of AA, helping millions of recovering addicts stay on the straight and narrow."

"How do you and the sponsor do it?" I asked.

"Just get in communication—share the hard days vulnerably, stay connected. We only hide when we're 'off the wagon' and ashamed."

Hiding and ashamed... that part resonated.

So, I asked Andreas to be my nail biting sponsor.

He said yes.

For the next three months we checked in almost daily. I'd send him photos of my nails (chewed or pristine); he encouraged me to keep going no matter what.

While I had a few slip ups, my nails and cuticles hadn't looked better for decades.

It was the accountability to him and admitting my imperfection ("I'm not going to beat this on my own") that helped me recognize the biting triggers and manage them.

I had won! Or so I had thought...

We completed our 60-day agreement and fell out of communication.

Shortly thereafter, I was off the no-nail-biting wagon and back to anxious chewing.

"Damnitt! I thought I had this thing beat—it's as if I've learned nothing."

Nine months and a particularly bad biting session later, I had had enough.

So, I started a Healthy Habits Challenge, this time also helping other people start or stop something for 100 days.

I set up a spreadsheet for all of us to track our progress, checking off a box indicating that we achieved our goal for the day (or not).

Some people aimed to stop or reduce drinking.

Some to stop smoking cigarettes.

Some to start walking every day.

Some to stop eating sweets.

I was amazed at our results:

One person went from two packs of smokes per day down to quitting.

One stopped drinking during the week (a real feat after drinking almost daily for years).

One did some sort of exercise every day...

I was really proud of the participants and myself—once again making good strides toward kicking the habit.

Shortly after the 100 Day Challenge, I reverted back to my old ways, stress-biting yet again.

"Ugh! What is wrong with me?!"

————— ∘ O ∘ —————

What I discovered after the second bout of success and failure is that I need continued support to not bite my nails. Regular, daily check-ins with someone. A sponsor.

So, I enrolled my friend (who gave up smoking in the Challenge) to be my daily sponsor. Cigarettes are a bitch to quit, so if he can overcome nicotine, I can certainly kick the nail-biting habit.

He simply checks in daily with a " 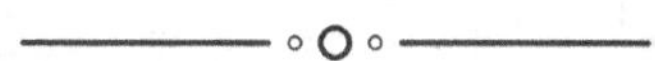 " emoji.

I respond with the number of days in my current streak of being bite-free.

And it works.

As of publishing this book, I've had the highest rate of success that I can remember.

Who knows what the future holds?

"Breath by breath," as they say in AA.

All I know from this experience is that accountability and partnership matter a lot when it comes to changing stubborn habits. A lot.

Have the courage to find support. Ask for help creating the life you want. That vulnerability? That's where your power comes from.

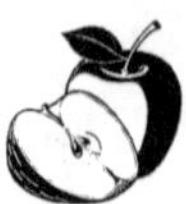

BOTTOM LINE:

- Sometimes we can change on our own. Sometimes we can't. And that's okay too. Knowing the difference is key.

- The point is that our shame, our shadow, comes to the light and starts to disappear when we're vulnerable enough to ask for support. And it allows others permission to do the same.

- If you're having difficulty kicking a habit (or starting one), I implore you to consider enlisting the support of a friend, a coach, a mentor, anyone you feel will hold you big and accountable.

- Maybe it's just for a few weeks or months. Maybe it's for a lifetime.

- Everything you've ever wanted to accomplish may just be a phone call away.

Push yourself physically at least once per week

> **Great things come from hard work and perseverance. No excuses.**
>
> - Kobe Bryant

"You looked at the clock again. So the round starts over. Begin... BEGIN!!!"

Tyler, my Muay Thai instructor, had had enough of me peeking at the clock during our conditioning drills.

It was a hot summer afternoon in a dank martial arts gym. Just me and him. I wished there were others he could focus on.

Tyler was a world champion kickboxer. He was so fluid, so accurate with his punches and kicks. He made Muay Thai look frustratingly easy.

I had picked up the sport a few months prior as a way to get in better shape and to learn self-defense.

I was fit, but not *this* type of fit. I was gym fit. 12 reps and rest fit. Not endless rounds of bag punching and kicking fit.

Deep down, I think he especially loved to see gym bros like me suffer.

On this day, Tyler wanted to see how deep I could dig. And I wasn't digging deep enough for his liking.

When fatiguing, I had this habit of looking at the dwindling round clock. Tyler picked up on it and made it a point to literally beat it out of me.

"Do the combination again. Jab. Jab. Hook. Cross. Slap kick. Knee Knee. Three times with the left then three times with the right. Go. GO!"

Jab. Jab. Hook. Knee... I screwed up his instruction again.

"WRONG! FOCUS!"

My terrible habit of clock-watching happened again... and Tyler caught me—again.

"START THE ROUND OVER. I've got all day for you to get this right."

This went on for literal minutes, but it felt like hours. I wouldn't know—I stopped looking at the clock.

When I finally did the combinations to his liking enough times, Tyler mercifully called the session. I was breathless, the mat covered in my sweat.

"Derek—champions win because they push themselves to the limit, not by waiting for the bell to ring. You'll discover how great you can be when you finally let your body overcome your mind."

I never forgot that lesson. "Go as long as I can, not as long as I think I can."

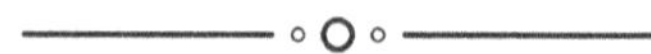

Think about it: when was the last time you really pushed yourself, physically?

I mean push-ups until your arms collapse... running as fast as you can... hiking up a vertical without stopping.

If you can't recall it within the last month (or year), it may be time to build this muscle again.

Long after I stopped training with Tyler, I still harken back to that day in that sweltering gym.

Don't get me wrong, training to abject failure every session is a recipe for injury and maladaptation, especially once we turn 30.

But an occasional dose of "push it!" goes a long way, with many benefits.

Prolonged training stimulus, increased lean body mass, cellular health, mental fortitude, longevity—our body adapts to the highest stimulus we place upon it, leaving us access to that newfound strength at a future workout, and often much more.

It goes without saying, high intensity training like this is the "habanero pepper" of the fitness foods—a little goes a long, long way. However, it can really make the dish.

Here's what I recommend when starting out:

Once per week, with a focus on precise form, push your body to its current limit.

There are many ways to achieve this:

- Four to eight 15-second sprints on a stationary bike or elliptical, done at the bottom of every minute with :45 rest in between

- One to two sets of strength training, such as push-ups or lunges, with two minutes of rest in between

- One plank, held as long as possible

- One wall sit, held as long as possible

- Run or walk a mile, as fast as possible

- Jump rope continuously until you mess up

It doesn't just have to be in the realm of exercise, either. Other ways to push your boundaries:

- Take the coldest shower possible

- Fast for 24+ hours

- Work on breath holds

Regardless of what you choose, elevate your efforts and push beyond current boundaries and beliefs. Record your progress (time or reps achieved) on a note in your phone or in a workout tracker/spreadsheet so you can beat it next week.

For the record, this is exactly how I did 100 push-ups in a row, ran a sub-six minute mile and performed 1,000 clean jumps in a row with a jump rope.

Nothing fancy, just a commitment to be a little better than the week before.

Some weeks I improved. Some weeks I didn't. Eventually I always achieved the objective.

It's uncomfortable. You may get sore for a couple of days in the beginning, depending on the activity. But the mental and physical benefits can't be found anywhere else in the training world.

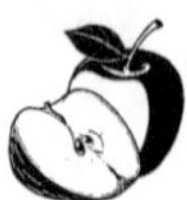

BOTTOM LINE:

- Short durations of peak effort create a powerful adaptation stimulus—benefitting fat loss, cardiovascular fitness, and cellular health.[6]

- A little maximal effort goes a long way, especially at the onset. Start with just one set of your chosen exercise to create a baseline and to build capacity safely.

- If engaging in a physical challenge, make sure to adequately warm up the muscles you'll be training with appropriate auxiliary exercises, movements, or preparations.

- Track your efforts to keep progress alive and in existence

Set yourself up for sleep success in the morning

> **Keep your face to the sunshine and you cannot see the shadows.**
>
> - Helen Keller

I was hung over.

Not college-level, keg-stands-and-bottom-shelf-vodka hungover (that would currently kill me), but a four-cocktail, out-until-12:30 hungover. Tired to the bone.

I wake up with that familiar ache behind my eyes—the gift of acetaldehyde, alcohol's toxic hangover-causing byproduct.

In spite of my plight, the kids are still up at 6:30am, and they don't care or understand the meaning of "hangover."

"Daddy, it's time to play Marie and Toothless," my daughter commands.

"Ugghhh."

I pretend not to hear her.

"Dadddyyyy."

Wifey gets to sleep in on the weekends—she is not coming to the rescue.

I rise slowly. Drink some water, splash cold water on my face.

And then I recall one of my favorite biohackers, Ben Greenfield, saying: "If you're tired in the morning, get outside in the early sun. Light is the most important stimulus for encouraging cortisol release and resetting circadian rhythm."

Big breath.

"Ok, Sophie—go get your dolls, throw a sweatshirt on, and meet me in the backyard."

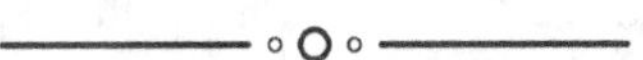

While sleep research began in the 19th century and sleep medicine was established as a field in the 1970s, our understanding of sleep's comprehensive role in health has exploded in the past two decades, with research now linking sleep to nearly every aspect of wellness.[7]

Other than food, there is no other singular factor more important to health than sleep.

Unfortunately, as we age it doesn't get any easier to come by! Do you remember your "sleeps" as a kid? I had flawless, immaculate rest all night and didn't think twice about it! Lucky bastard...

Here's what happens: Melatonin and GABA—the hormones that help you sleep and stay calm—decline as you age. Throw in life stress, nobody telling you to go to bed, and whatever bad habits you picked up in your twenties. Result? You can't fall asleep. You can't stay asleep. And you're definitely not getting quality rest.

But all is not lost! We can re-learn how to rest, and it actually begins with our actions in the morning, as well as throughout the day leading up to bedtime.

Here are a few practices to implement, from sunup to sundown:

Wake up easy: I use a sleep tracker that quietly buzzes on my wrist to wake me. I'll never go back to a blaring alarm—especially after having a baby in our room when I needed to wake without disturbing anyone else. If you don't want to invest in a sleep tracker (like an Oura Ring or Apple Watch), there are haptic alarm bracelets on Amazon for a fraction of the cost. Another option: alarm clocks that wake you with slowly intensifying light and sound to mimic sunrise and nature sounds. Search "sunrise alarm clock" on Google or Amazon.

Get morning sun to reset your circadian rhythm: Rays from the rising sun suppress lingering effects of melatonin. Get a dose of it upon waking to shake off any sleep residue. The sun is less severe at this time, so hang out a few minutes and don't worry about getting a sunburn. Bonus points for moving your lymphatic system by walking or adding a few stretches while catching the rays. Extra movement in the morning will also start to stimulate your first bowel movement *sans* coffee.

Water upon waking: Resist the urge to go right to the coffee pot and hydrate with 16 ounces of pure, mineral-rich water first. This will help flush out accumulated toxins with a morning pee or two and continue to wake up the digestive tract without stimulants.

Coffee after water: Did you know our naturally-rising cortisol helps prepare us for waking in the morning? Our circadian rhythm has cortisol levels peaking around 7-8am. Some experts suggest that coffee as a pick-me-up might be more effective after that peak— around 9:30-11am when cortisol levels decline—though research on optimal timing is still limited and individual responses vary.[8]

Skip the afternoon cup: If you get jittery and anxious after one cup of coffee, skip the second one. Caffeine stimulates the adrenal system, releasing cortisol with effects that can linger 6-10 hours and interrupt sleep.[9] Depending on your ability to metabolize caffeine (with the enzyme cytochrome P450 1A2), you may just want to keep intake as early as possible.[10] If you must have a second one, take it with L-theanine, an amino acid which can help smooth out the jitters.[11] Green tea has both caffeine and l-theanine, so a good compromise beverage there.

Have a late afternoon snack of carbohydrates and cheese: A health book recommending carbs and cheese?! Seriously. Carbohydrates boost serotonin production which aids in sleep. Cheese is filling which will help you eat less at dinner, which typically also aids in improving sleep. Just don't overdo the portion size! A palmful of carbohydrates and a thumb or two of cheese is plenty.

Wrap up work 2-3 hours before bed: A combination of work stress, blue light from screens, and not enough downtime will prevent you from falling asleep (melatonin suppression and sleep latency), and getting quality sleep (increased pulse rate and decreased heart rate variability).

Exercise at least three hours before bed: Exercise—especially cardio—creates "good stress" (eustress) that can keep you wired for hours. Your nervous system stays in "fight or flight" mode long after you're done.

If evenings are your only workout window, avoid high-intensity stuff like spin class. Better choices: strength training (you probably need more of this anyway—great for aging hormones), gentle yoga, walking. Save the intense workouts for weekends when you have recovery time.

Food 2-3 hours away from sleep: Pending the size of meal, your body dedicates about 10% of daily energy to digestion.[12]

If you eat right before bed, your digestive organs aren't focused on resting and clearing but processing food later into the night. Make lunch your biggest meal and pare down dinner.

Alcohol and adult substances 3–4 hours before sleep: Ladies, keep it to one drink; fellas, one to two (but gotta tell ya—the drop-off in sleep quality after even one is precipitous... less is more here). Marijuana and its tetrahydrocannabinol component (THC, the psychoactive part of the plant) can disrupt REM sleep—the brain-supporting kind.[13] While some find it helps them fall asleep, I've experienced the opposite and personally steer clear of evening imbibement.

Shower with hot and cold contrasting water 1-2 hours before bed:

The vasodilation and vasoconstriction of our blood vessels from alternating hot and cold water before bed can promote restfulness. Start warm, followed by a few seconds of cold-as-you-can-take water, alternating a spell of hot. Repeat a few times, finishing with hot.

Turn off TV/screens 1-2 hours before bed: While any blaring screen can disrupt sleep onset, I find high-drama TV shows particularly stimulating before bed. If you watch crime shows and find it hard to relax afterwards, maybe just stick with some Brady Bunch or Love On The Spectrum reruns. If you must look at a screen leading up to bed, be sure to dim its brightness as much as possible. You can also seek out "night-time" mode on your device, which will reduce screen blare, and won't flood your brain with melatonin-suppressing blue light.

Prepare for the next day 0-1 hours before bed: Clear your head with a to-do list. Set clothes out, prep your food and water. Leave nothing floating about your mind so rest comes with as much ease as possible.

Give love to your friends and family before bed: Long hugs, kisses and cuddles release oxytocin, which counteracts stress and anxiety and fosters relaxation. If you don't have someone to do that with at home, a phone call or text expressing love and gratitude can also create a sense of well-being and social connection.

Putting these pieces together may take time—perhaps you'll just want to start with getting a little sunshine in the morning or drinking a little water before coffee. Wherever you begin, all will make incremental differences toward improved sleep quality and quantity. Become masterful at these steps, and sleep will once again become second nature.

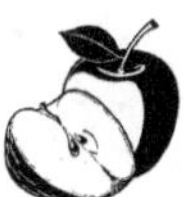

BOTTOM LINE:

- For many (including myself), good sleep doesn't happen as easily as it used to.

- Use these practices and stick to these timeframes to get the best sleep possible. It starts the moment you wake up.

- Start small, start now.

- Visit **eattheapplebook.com** to download your sleep success guide.

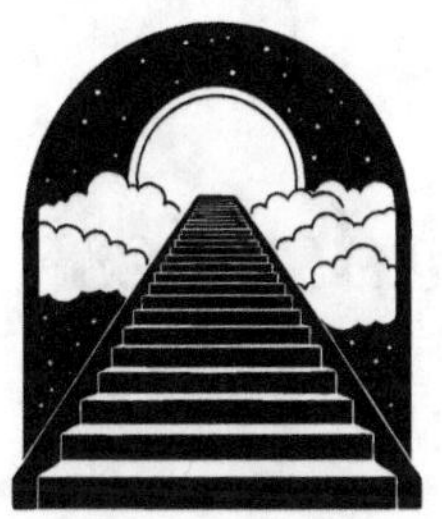

FINAL FLIGHT

More "ands," less "buts"

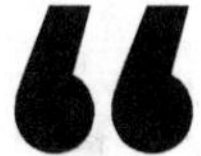

> # As I say yes to life, life says yes to me.
>
> – Louise Hay

"I want to be healthier and look better. As a gay man, this is even more crucial... but I'm just so busy! I'm absolutely swamped at the office, then I've got to jump on Zoom for a monthly board meeting at 6:30, followed by dinner plans for a friend's birthday at 9:00. And this is my life all the time! Outside of seeing you each week, how the hell can I fit anything else in?!"

Russel is... busy.

He gives much of his time and money to animal rights and adoption groups, has lots of friends who like to hang out with him (especially because he's a culturephile that knows all of LA's best restaurants). When he's not in LA, he's traveling for work or pleasure, but always working even if it's pleasure.

Russel's winning in life by most accounts. At a surface level, his reasons for not prioritizing healthy habits are valid. Work. Charitable giving. A large group of friends.

But... he's 40 pounds overweight. Unhealthy for anyone, but especially troublesome as an urban gay male with the added cultural stigma.

But... his health suffers. He's stressed, stuck at his desk without enough movement. No planning ahead with food leaves him starving—then bingeing when he finally eats. Too many late nights, late meals, and late drinks mean poor sleep 3-5 nights per week. He never gets the chance to unplug and recover.

But... most challenging of all, he doesn't see how to shift the life he leads without giving up everything and starting life all over.

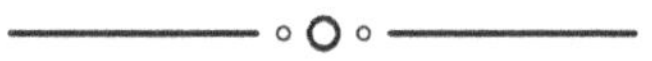

Russel's case is not an extraordinary one. I've heard some version of it so many times. Perhaps you, too, have been infected with a bad case of the "buts."

"I'd like to find time to exercise, but I'm just too busy."

"I'd like to get more sleep, but I want to watch my shows before bed."

"I'd like to eat more vegetables, but I just don't like the taste."

"But" is a sneaky little word. Have a deeper look.

If you break a "but" statement down into parts, the words preceding the "but" speak into a new future of possibility. It's typically something we might want to achieve or change about ourselves and our practices. Something distinct and better than we've got right now.

However, the words following "but" pull us back into our present reality, removing the possibility of moving forward with the initial desire—and keep us stuck where we don't necessarily want to be anymore.

Saying "but" after expressing a desire first is like arguing for being right when you don't want to be right. "But" puts a foot on the brake while the other is on the gas.

And when we blame a circumstance outside of oneself for the results we're getting (or not getting), it costs us vitality, self-expression, and ultimately the outcomes we want.

Saying "but" makes whatever you said after it final and non-negotiable. And we don't want that.

The easiest way I've found to cure myself of the "buts" is to do a little word magic.

First, simply flip the statements before and after the "but" then put an "and" in its place instead.

For example, change: "I want to lose weight, but I don't have time to exercise."

To: "I don't have time to exercise, and I want to lose weight."

After the statement, add the word "so," indicating there's more opportunity coming.

"I don't have time to exercise, and I want to lose weight, so I've got to find 10 minutes each morning to do push-ups and make a smoothie."

"And/so" statements open our brains up to the world of possibility again. Instead of being stuck in the "what is currently true" of our present reality, we allow our brain's anterior lateral prefrontal cortex to look for conceivable alternatives within our environment to have the results in spite of the perceived reality.

As legendary entrepreneur Henry Ford famously said: "Whether you think you can, or you think you can't, you are right."

Let language be a sail, not an anchor, when it comes to moving toward your desired outcomes.

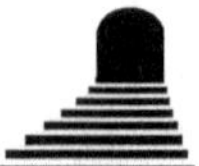

BOTTOM LINE:

- Blaming busyness for lack of results makes you ineffective. Don't get frustrated, get curious.

- When desiring a different lifestyle outcome yet feeling stuck, take a moment to check the language you're speaking—it's the critical foundation of change.

- When thinking negatively or small ("but I can't" statements), perform a little word magic: Speak the last part first, the first part last, switch out the "but" for an "and," then add a "so" at the end, followed by an action that will forward you toward the desired outcome.

Joie de vivre—Finding a joy for life (and health) again

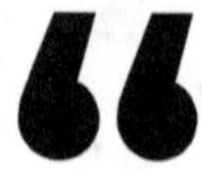

> **The most beautiful moments in life are moments when you are expressing joy, not when you are seeking it.**
>
> - Sadhguru

My mom said I was born happy.

The first day my parents took me home from the hospital I slept through the night. When I could barely walk, I grabbed a comb, climbed on my grandparents' sofa, and mimicked the happy-go-lucky Sesame Street game show host "Guy Smiley" for my family.

Growing up, I loved to do vocal impressions of my favorite TV and movie characters. I loved to laugh and make people laugh. I always had teachers cracking up (no doubt turning some of those C+'s into B's).

But as I grew older some of that ease and play faded. I got popular. I got better looking. I got validation for something other than my humor and happiness. And it took some of my joy away.

Fast forward to 30 years old...

Opening my first gym studio, having an unexpected pregnancy with someone I just started dating, feeling the weight to be a "provider"... something changed as the burdens and expectations of adulthood grew heavy.

Kids and bills and retirement planning took even more of the natural luster off my sunny disposition.

"You're not as funny as you used to be," my mom told me during a visit home from California some years ago, before my first child was born. "There's a seriousness about you that wasn't there before."

Joslyn, my girlfriend and future mother of my child at the time, would say: "Are you okay? I know you've got a lot on your plate but you're so distant. I miss that funny boy."

After I eschewed yet another invite to hang out, my best friend Frankie said, "Don't forget your friends, homie—we want to support you but can't if you avoid us."

I wanted to say "No duh—I'm drowning over here—have you seen my life lately?"

But beyond the obvious challenges, they all were right. As much as I was already sliding away from my innate happiness, I was relating to this newfound adulthood especially poorly.

I had begun focusing so much on surviving my life, I wasn't enjoying any of it, and my way of being was impacting those I loved.

After a particularly pointed fight with Joslyn about my way of being I knew I had to change something. My relationship depended on it.

During my ride into work the next morning, I thought, "There's so much to love about life, hectic as it can be. It's time to do something... be something different."

I slowly started to step out of my fog and consciously looked for moments that made me joyful, funny, grateful, excited, curious, connected again.

I made time for walks with my pregnant girlfriend. I made sure to send little digital cards to clients showing my appreciation for them. I had heart to heart conversations repairing the relationships I had neglected. I leaned into my Jar of Awesome. I thanked God every morning. I found podcasts with speakers that uplifted my spirit. I caught myself taking things too seriously and changed course (or at least eventually did). I looked up at the night sky and enjoyed the stars.

It's easy to sum up the shift in a few paragraphs, but it truly took time and effort to return to joy. And it definitely wasn't a clean, linear walk up the mountain to nirvana.

There are a myriad things about work and parenthood to complain about. Anything for that matter. Dickhead bosses. Sleepless babies with diaper rash. Stressful commutes.

And as Viktor Frankl says in A Man's Search for Meaning: "Everything can be taken from a man but one thing: the last of the human freedoms—to choose one's attitude in any given set of circumstances, to choose one's own way."

And it can be done.

My little hack lately to check in with my internal state is to simply step out of my default thinking and ask (internally or aloud), "*Joie?*"

As in—"Am I experiencing 'Joy' just because I can choose it?"

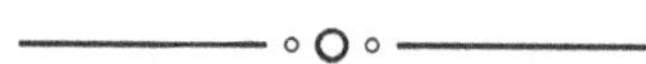

So much of our happiness is a concerted choice.

In the wise words of Eleanor Roosevelt, "When you change the way you look at things, the things you look at change."

I'm constantly wanting more: more material success, more status, more impact. I struggle to be satisfied with all the inherent and created abundance I've got in the present moment

"Capricorns: perpetually dissatisfied," an astrologer once told me at a holiday party (I'm a textbook Capricorn, born January 3rd).

Even someone with a generally sunny disposition like me wrestles with wanting more than I currently have in the realm of finance, physique development, beauty—it goes on and on.

The people with the most money, the most beauty, the most homes, the most travel? They'll be the first to tell you: none of it matters if you refuse to be happy with what you have.

I think it is human nature to desire an elevated station in life, and generally a good thing to have ambition for more. Yet, with perpetual desires burning in the background, it can be hard to recognize the sweet, joyful moments available all around us.

And they're ever-present! I consider these reasons to be joyful on a macroscale:

Living in America or another developed country is something to give great thanks for—millions of immigrants around the world would give nearly anything to live where I live.

A roof over my head—many millions of global citizens don't have that.

Gainful employment that allows my family the resources so my wife doesn't have to work, and she's free to raise our children on our terms.

Deep, intimate relationships with friends—many of whom I've known for over 20 and 30 years.

Healthy food and clean water... clean air to breathe.

Life-enhancing books to read and courses to take.

Beyond these, living life with "*Joie*" means appreciating small things in the present moment:

That first sip of coffee in the morning. Chewing our food slowly. Basking in the sunshine. The smell and beauty of a flower. Appreciating the embrace from a loved one. Greeting a happy baby after their nap.

In other words, *joie de vivre* is to savor the experience of our experience.

From that vantage point, it's easy to see how rich we are!

And it is contagious. Embody joy for others, and choose to be around those who embody joy. In a world of "I'm not enough," it's an essential way of being that attracts more of the same.

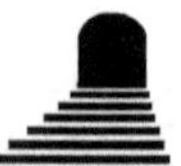

BOTTOM LINE:

- Joy for living is a moment by moment choice.

- Material wealth means nothing without appreciation for it.

- Start by appreciating the big things, then focus on the small ones as you develop your *joie*.

- A joyful outlook spreads easily, and attracts more of the same.

A little bit of cold

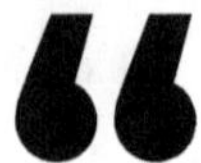

> **If we had no winter, the spring would not be so pleasant.**
>
> - Anne Bradstreet

"Get naked. And get in the water."

It was the final night of my first coaching program intensive.

"Nope. Nope. Not going in there."

Four months of life-transforming challenges and experiences. I hated it. I wanted to quit every minute of it. I was perpetually uncomfortable for the entire experience (and creating myriad breakthroughs).

And like twisting a dagger into me (and all of my fellow participants), the head instructor had one last plunge up their sleeve.

"Cold water signifies a cleansing of the mind and body. A completion of the past, bringing clarity to your future. There are few things more confronting than this experience. You're cold. You'll soon be naked. You thought we were here just to send you off with a pat on the back? You've made it this far. This is your opportunity to take on everything that's weighed you down in the past and leave it in the lake. To get everything you desire, life will continue to require bold, uncomfortable experiences like this one. Jump in and discover just how amazing you'll feel after you do... or don't, and wonder 'what-if.'"

I and the other students waffled on the dock for a moment until a participant just said, "Hell with it," stripped off her clothes, and ran for the water.

I and others quickly followed, stripping down to nothing, laying it all out in the cool summer air.

I chose to cannonball in.

The 60-degree Lake Arrowhead water took my breath away. For a moment it consumed me and I was left in shock. I found myself gasping and flapping in the water, unsure of how else to respond but with guttural modulations.

I sprinted to the shore.

"Stay there!" our coach commanded.

"Stay in the water and be with it! Be with all of it!"

She calmed her intensity to try and calm ours.

"Breathe... calm your body and breathe into the sensation. Find your breath here and you can find it through anything. For thirty more seconds, I ask you to be there now."

Those of us who could stand it did our best to breathe and... just be. For a brief moment, I calmed my mind enough to block out the pain and capture the essence of what she meant... to access an inner calm that is always available, no matter the external locus.

The time is up. We get to shore, towels awaiting... accomplishment achieved.

I'd like to think I've experienced the euphoria of doing some pretty joy-inducing events in my life. Seeing the birth of my children, delivering a keynote speech, skydiving, beating the rival school in sports...

And outside of my kids being born, nothing has come close to the natural high I attained jumping in that cold lake. Nothing.

We get back to the lodge, comfy sweats on, warmed by the fire, waiting for food to be served.

"We did it, dude... we did it," my friend and fellow participant Radcliffe said, each of us basking in the moment after the final mission was complete.

"We did. This will be a night I will never forget."

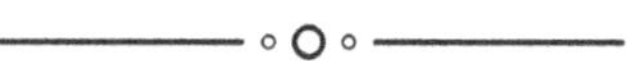

Up until that night, I had never completed a coaching course. I was truly elated to take on my life and experience so many breakthroughs in four short months. After jumping in the lake, I experienced a mushroom trip-level of ecstasy (the magical kind of mushroom, not the one in your salad).

It was also the first time I had ever voluntarily jumped into cold, cold water like that and intentionally experienced the effects.

At the time, I attributed my unbridled joy solely to completing the rigorous course. I've done many courses since then (without plunging into cold water afterwards), and none matched that peak feeling.

No, in hindsight the secret sauce to elation was the cold water.

As a young personal trainer at the time, I was conceptually aware of the benefits of cold immersion but was in no rush to find my nearest lake and experience the "benefits" myself.

Hell, I'm not sure I ever even took a cool shower up to that point!

Aside from that realization, I never picked up the practice until years later, during a health coaching course that extolled the virtues of cold-water immersion and encouraged us to experience it firsthand.

When I started to make it a practice (slowly, gently), I immediately felt the benefits.

Here's how short term cold exposure supports some of our systems from a 10,000 foot view:

Brain health: Cold exposure increases RBM3 (cold-shock proteins) and catecholamines—or hormones that are produced in response to stress (such as norepinephrine, dopamine, and epinephrine—which are crucial to "synaptic plasticity," an important function to maintain learning and memory pathways.

Fat loss: Olympic gold medalist Michael Phelps famously consumed 8,000-10,000 calories daily during peak training—not the widely-reported but mythical 12,000.[1] He used ice baths as part of his recovery routine. Separately, breathwork guru Wim "The Iceman" Hof—who trekked partway up Mt. Everest wearing only basketball shorts[2]—claims cold exposure (and the regulatory mechanisms involved with shivering and non-shivering thermogenesis) boosts metabolism by over 15%.

Increased immunity: The old saying, "You'll catch a cold in the cold" turns out to be partly true. Cold weather can make it easier to catch a virus. Your nasal passages cool down. Immune defenses drop. Viruses have an easier time getting in. But here's the twist: deliberate cold exposure—cold showers, ice baths—might actually help. The shock triggers stress hormones that mobilize white blood cells.[3] It's controlled stress. Training your body's response systems. Not a cure-all, but a signal to your immune system to stay sharp.

Mood booster: No surprise to me here. Cold exposure releases noradrenaline—a jolt of alertness that activates your nervous system. The cold receptors in your skin send electrical impulses to your brain, potentially boosting mood and motivation.[4] Some researchers think cold showers might help with depression, though the evidence is still early.[5] The catch: cold exposure temporarily impairs cognition, affecting memory and reaction time during and after exposure. Know the trade-offs.

I realize it may take more than stats and process explanations to get someone to jump in a cold lake. Unless you're training to be a Navy SEAL, I wouldn't recommend that as a starting point for nearly anyone.

Seriously, the shift in temperature can be such a shock to the system it can threaten paralysis, heart failure, and drowning. That is NOT the place to begin this kind of journey.

However, the many benefits of cold immersion can be introduced safely and simply from the (relative) comfort of your own home.

Here's how I've managed to build cold tolerance into my wellness regimen:

Beginner: Fill up your bathroom wash basin with the coldest water possible. Add ice cubes if not cold enough. Hold your breath and immerse your face (which has the highest amount of sensory receptors in the whole body) for 15-30 seconds. Repeat 2-3x. This is the easiest and most effective segue into the cold immersion realm!

Moderate options:

Alternating shower: Jump in the shower as the water turns on, making sure to soak the entire body. Let water warm up for a spell. Continue to alternate temperature down and up 3-5x.

Cool/Cold shower: Turn on the shower and get in while the water is still warming up—keep water temperature at the coolest setting you can manage. If you're doing this in the evening, complete the shower with warm/hot water for a relaxing finish. Dilating and constricting the vascular system can be a safe and natural sleep aide.

Cold shower: Keep water as cold as you can manage for the duration of the session. Even a few short seconds can start to provide mood and energy boosting benefits! I will sometimes just go between having cold water and off/no water at all, sudsing up and washing off my body and hair in the dry periods, rinsing off my bits with the cold. A true California water saver!

Advanced: Fill up the tub with cold water and 30-50 lbs ice and soak your body. Maybe you just start with the waist. Then the chest. Then bobbing head in and out. Start with 1-2 minutes, building from there.

Suggestion for all options: Breath and body control are the keys to mastering cold immersion—notice everything your body is doing in response to the stimulus: holding/shortening breath, tightening up body parts, clenching jaws or fists.

Progress to the next level only once you can manage body and breath control with an easier version.

Start with short durations—build capacity and tolerance.

Notice how you genuinely feel after the immersion is complete. My experience has always been refreshed, vibrant, alert... if you're employing this in the evening, I suggest curbing the energy boost with a warm/hot water finish to encourage restfulness.

Cold immersion is great for those who need a morning or afternoon burst of energy. The quality and duration of cognitive boost beats coffee every time.

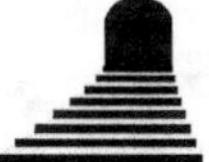

BOTTOM LINE:

- A few short minutes of cold exposure yields many physical, mental, and emotional benefits.

- Start on the easy end and build tolerance.

- Start with once a week, building up to cold exposure a few times per week.

Just a few supplements
Good ones

> **Supplements can't make up for a poor diet, but they can enhance a good one.**
>
> - Derek Opperman

Josh raised an eyebrow during our first call. "A smoothie, huh? Not usually what I do for breakfast. Not so sure about this 'nutritional powder' you're recommending, either."

It was his wife who contacted me about creating a health coaching program—Josh was 'voluntold' he'd also be participating.

He was right to be resistant. As a successful entrepreneur and family man, there wasn't a ton of extra bandwidth for Josh to add new habits. Any proposed change had to be easily integrated and noticeably effective.

"I was skeptical, too, at first," I said. "I thought a smoothie couldn't hold a candle to my bacon and eggs, and many protein powders up to that point left me gassy and bloated."

"Exactly," Josh affirmed.

"Allow me to show you the difference between your typical protein powder and the one I'm recommending you put in your smoothie."

I went on to show him side-by-side labels of the standard protein powder and the nutritional powder with protein.

- One has a complete dose of your daily vitamin and mineral needs, the other doesn't

- One is major allergen free; the other isn't

- One is cold processed to preserve protein quality; the other is heat-treated

- Both are complete proteins

- One is third party tested; the other would rather not say.

"On top of these distinctions, I like this product because the vitamins and minerals sourced are top quality—no cheap fillers here."

Josh was starting to see that not all supplements are created equal.

"Tell you what—try on this smoothie practice using the recommended nutritional support powder for the month. If you don't feel a distinct physical improvement, I'll eat my words and you can go back to coffee and a bagel."

Josh contemplated...

"Okay, deal."

Four years later, Josh starts his day with a smoothie using the same nutritional support powder I recommended back then.

"My work and travel schedule can be unpredictable. Crazy at times," he says, "And I need to be on top of my game. But one foundational habit I've instilled is that no matter where I'm going, I pack my daily nutritional support powder to ensure breakfast is handled. I can literally feel the difference if I don't use it."

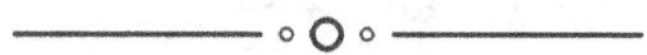

The supplement industry has exploded. Two decades ago? Ex-hippies at specialty stores selling vitamins. Now? A $193 billion industry growing 9% every year.[6]

However, because there is no governing body to verify efficacy claims supplement companies make, the industry is rife with snake oils and cheap substitutes.

Be on the lookout for these red flags:

- **Proprietary blend:** Means a company isn't disclosing how much of each ingredient is in the supplement—this is a red flag!

- **No expiration date:** Quality supplements have clearly marked expiration dates. If you can't find one, or if it looks suspicious, skip that product.

Labels to look for:

Since there is no government oversight to verify manufacturer claims, quality companies will source a third party group to test their products and ensure they have the ingredients they say they do, in the amounts listed.

Look for these certification labels:

GMP (Good Manufacturing Practices): Ensures the manufacturing facility follows FDA guidelines for quality, safety, and consistency.

USP (United States Pharmacopeia): Third party testing of vitamins, minerals, fish oils, glucosamine, and melatonin products. Ensures products contain the ingredients listed on their label at levels listed, don't contain harmful levels of contaminants, and will be bioavailable.

NSF (National Sanitation Foundation): Verifies that the ingredients listed are actually in the product, is tested for contaminants and that manufacturing facilities meet quality and safety standards.

NSF + Certified Sport: The most rigorous testing certification. Products are tested for 290 banned substances such as stimulants and anabolics. Rules out heavy metals, microorganisms, pesticides, and herbicides.

While everyone's bioindividual needs are different, these are a few foundational supplements I take regularly:

Daily Nutritional Support: Daily multivitamin, minerals, and 20 grams of plant-based, hypoallergenic protein—my favorite is EquiLife.

Fish oil/Omega 3: Supports brain, heart, and circulatory health. Look for triglyceride or phospholipid based (not ester based), held in a dark bottle to protect from oxidation, and high EPA/DHA content (not just total fish oil).

Fruit and Vegetable powder: Helps fill nutritional gaps in the diet. While NOT a replacement for actual fruits and vegetables, it's quick to prepare, travels well, and encourages hydration. Seek out certified organic and third party tested labels. Brands I like—VitalBody, Zena, and Organifi.

Creatine: By far the most researched supplement in the world for athletic performance. Essential for building and maintaining muscle, especially for women who strength train. Start with a quarter dose to assess tolerance.

Amino Acids: Protein in its simplest, most usable form. Look for a label that says "essential" amino acids. Great to use during workouts, when cutting calories, or during extended fasts.

Outside of those, I'll occasionally take:

- Zinc, elderberry, echinacea, oregano oil, and L-lysine if feeling under the weather

- Berberine and digestive enzymes if having a cheat day

- DHM (dihydromyricetin) if drinking alcohol to mitigate hangovers

- Liver support with milk thistle, n-acetyl-cysteine, and dandelion root when doing an extended fast.

While supplements can be supportive, it should go without saying that whole foods come first. Supplements are supplements—they fill gaps, not plates.[7]

We get so much more beyond vitamins and minerals with food. We need to chew for oral health, satiety signaling, and digestive enzyme production.

However, due to soil degradation from mass mono-agriculture and, in turn, a severe loss of nutrients from those practices, taking a few supplements to shore up deficiencies can be appropriate.

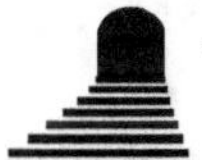

BOTTOM LINE:

- Taking a few quality certified supplements can shore up any dietary nutritional deficiencies and have us feeling our best.

- Look for third party certifications (GMP, USP, NSF) to ensure quality and safety.

- Supplements support a healthy diet—they don't replace one.

Make your CHO schedule

> # Yes of course, who has time... who has time? But then, if we do not take time, how can we ever have time?

— Merovingian, The Matrix Reloaded

"Hey D., can we move our second session to Friday at 6:00 next week?"

Mark asked after a training session.

"I think so—everything okay?" I asked.

"Yes, crazy week ahead. I've got a call with Warner Brothers on my calendar to renegotiate our upcoming contract, and I've got to prepare with my team for the panel I'm leading in Paris next Friday afternoon at our usual training time."

"Oh wow. Okay, let me check. Yes, we can train at 6:00 AM next week," I said, confirming the time change.

"Okay, thanks... just seeing it's also Lucille's school drama production that afternoon," he noted aloud, after scanning the calendar on his phone again.

"Busy week!"

"Always. My calendar is a living, breathing representation of my life—not sure how I'd manage all this in my head."

Mark is a hard charging executive vice president of a digital analytics company. He's also married with two young children. If anybody knows how important it is to schedule out a busy life, it's him.

"Sounds like you're managing three calendars at once."

"You'd think! But no, not lately. Before I got married and sold my company, it was really just a party of one—I didn't need to rely on a calendar to help me keep track of my work, family, and well-being. But once I got hitched and hired by a company, life became too big not to integrate all of life's aspects in one place. Doubly so, when kids came around. It all has to work or nothing will work."

"Do you plan out your well-being, too?"

"That's the first thing I schedule!" he said excitedly. "My calendar is really the first barometer of my health game and living a semblance of a balanced life. If I start to miss workouts, runs, or lose sleep from late meetings, I know I'm doing too much and will catch a cold that takes me out for two weeks."

"Yikes—who knew a calendar could be such an essential tool?" I mused.

"You're telling me. Okay, gotta run and get the kids to school. See? It's in the calendar, right there," Mark said with a wink.

"Indeed it is—see you next week at 6:00!"

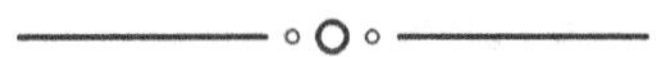

Here's something you may or may not know: CEOs of companies live and die by their calendar. They must write everything down that needs to get done (and by when), or the organization they run will become dysfunctional or inefficient.

As Chief Health Officer of your body, implementing meaningful habits long term requires a schedule to remember and perform the regular actions that keep a body trim, vibrant, and confident in perpetuity.

If you've got a "there's not enough time to be healthy" conversation going on in your brain, or say, "I know what I should be doing, I just don't do it," a lot, then creating your CHO schedule can be a game-changer.

Building your CHO schedule is simple:

Sit down with your calendar open—paper or digital—before the start of your week.

Fill out your calendar as normal—work and family obligations, social events, phone calls... get it all down. Speak with your partner and make sure nothing else is missing.

Once you've squeezed everything out and have got it down to clearly see, look for the 5-60 minute gaps between the time you wake up and the time you go to bed...

What are you noticing? I find most people are amazed by the gaps they actually have—not always huge blocks of time (though sometimes that, too!) but small pockets of opportunity to weave more health into their busy lives without even realizing it.

While a full gym or food prep session can sometimes be fit in, there are often smaller opportunities available to access well-being when we look for them.

- Break between meetings? Get outside or make time to move.

- Feeling peckish? Whip up a greens drink instead of reaching for a bag of potato chips.

- Don't have a particularly busy day? Consider doing a modified fast.

- Crushed the sales meeting, had a great performance review, or the head of the PTA paid you a compliment? Add it to your Jar of Awesome.

When you find available space or discover an already-scheduled task that can be "stacked" upon, insert your health action that fits into the time slot.

Visual hack: Use a different colored writing utensil or tag to denote the health-centric habits you'd like to implement (it really works! Thank your brain's posterior midline cortex for that). This way, you'll be able to quickly remind yourself of the actions you intend to take that are distinct from work and social obligations.

When applicable, the CHO schedule is a great way to share our health practices with partners or buddies—even better, enroll them onto your health team and share tasks for accountability.

If you've got some consistency in schedule, set the habit reminder on repeat so it's set week after week. This is also nice because the habit stays on the schedule, so you can move it around a bit if life throws a curveball.

If there are multiple steps (such as a habit stack or routine), lay out your habit(s) in the notes section within the reminder (for example—nighttime routine—7:30pm—make smoothies, pack lunch, refill water bottles + add electrolytes, pick tomorrow's outfit and shoes, etc.).

Finally, set one or more alarms to remind you to perform the action—this keeps the practice alive, especially in those early days when you're building new habits. Keep them front and center, or they'll slip away before they stick.

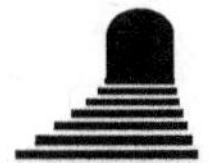

BOTTOM LINE:

- Busy as we are, there's always an opportunity to optimize our available time.

- Schedule your week as normal and after that's complete, find the 5-60 minute openings throughout—this book will help you fill in those gaps with most-effective practices.

- Color code your health-related habits.

- Share your health habits calendar with a partner, friend, or accountability buddy.

- Schedule your habits on repeat with alarm reminders until they're ingrained.

Keep Your Commitments While Traveling

> **One's destination is never a place, but a new way of seeing things.**
>
> - Henry Miller

After another exhausting week on the road, Jerry returned home feeling a sharp tightness in his chest—a persistent pressure he could no longer ignore.

The prior months had been a blur of planes, trains, and rental cars. Lavish lunches, indulgent dinners, countless cocktails—all part of the endless cycle of entertaining clients. Late nights blurred into early flights.

His body was sending a message.

"I confided in my father-in-law, a doctor. He wasted no time taking me to the hospital."

Jerry was kept overnight. A heart catheterization was performed the next morning.

"My blood work revealed pre-diabetes, dangerously high cholesterol, and the need for heart medication. This was definitely one of those 'come to Jesus' moments."

"I was forced to take a hard look at my life—the toll my habits and career had taken."

At 46, Jerry had built a beautiful life. Loving family. Thriving career. But his lifestyle had brought him here.

"I hadn't been thinking beyond today—toward being present for my children."

These days, Jerry's mornings and evenings begin with eight to nine medications—managing blood sugar, cholesterol, atrial fibrillation, acid reflux, arteriosclerosis, spinal pain.

"It feels like there's always another trip to CVS."

Looking back, I can't help but wonder: Could Jerry have prevented this? If he'd adopted a leaner diet, cut back on alcohol, sought a less demanding career—would he be in a better place today?

Now he's playing catch-up, working to undo years of damage.

Nevertheless, life carries on.

"I'm learning to embrace this new normal, to accept my limitations. Yet I can't ignore that this reality is a direct result of choices I made in the past."

—————— ∘ O ∘ ——————

I've seen travel derail health plans more times than I like to admit.

There's something about being on the road that has people throw their hands up: "Nothing I can do! I'll start over when I get home."

Yet many find it hard to get back into routine after even a few days away.

If we don't interrupt this cycle, travel will almost assuredly include:

- Unpredictable food

- Increased alcohol

- Unfamiliar beds / irregular sleep

- Packed schedules

- Days indoors breathing recirculated air

- Time changes and jet lag

It really takes something to overcome this inertia.

But cracking this code is how we have the health and body we want—anywhere, anytime.

Here are a few questions to answer before your next trip:

- Where to? How long?

- Time zone changes?

- Staying in a hotel, AirBnB, or with family?

- Urban, rural, or remote?

- Access to grocery stores and restaurants?

- Will alcohol be present/encouraged? How many occasions?

- Is there a gym? Does it have weights?

Once I've got a dignified look at those components, I can develop a strategy.

Here's how:

Food:

Airport food is notoriously unhealthy and expensive, so I always pack food for the first flight and a few days of snacks—especially if grocery stores aren't within walking distance.

Travel-friendly options I like:

- Apples and peanut butter packets (Justin's brand)

- Carrots, celery and individual hummus containers

- Raw nuts and raisins

- Protein bars (minimally processed, few ingredients)

- Grass-fed jerky sticks

Bonus points for packing a small soft cooler with an ice pack—keeps food fresh and prevents squishing.

I research restaurants in advance to find healthy options. Google, Yelp, and Tripadvisor are good starting points.

Fitness:

If staying in a hotel: Does it have a gym? Weights?

If not, I bring 2-3 exercise bands. They weigh nothing and pack into a running shoe.

Check out local trails or green spaces nearby.

Pack running shoes for local discovery or at least a treadmill session.

Sleep:

I bring a sleep mask to ensure decent rest no matter where I am or which way the window faces.

Earplugs or white noise from my phone (I like "rolling warm dryer") to drown out errant noise.

Alcohol:

Know thyself and thy work/leisure culture.

Whether vacation or work, see how much alcohol and late nights are woven through the trip. If drinking is expected and you want to imbibe, stay dry before traveling and get quality rest the week prior—be proactive with your liver and enjoy the party more when it happens.

Even better: Hit the happy hour early and taper off. Alcohol has the greatest impact on sleep quality. The further your consumption is from bedtime, the better your rest (up to an extent—more than three or four cocktails and you're screwed either way).

Stick to clear liquors to mitigate hangover potential. Anything brown or red is fermented more, producing higher levels of congeners and histamines (which make hangovers worse).

If you're concerned with the optics of not partaking (abstaining from poison at social events is an offensive paradox to some people), switch to club soda with a splash of cranberry and lime after one or two - no one will notice.

Agenda:

If traveling for a work conference, take every opportunity to get outside.

Go for a walk/run in the morning before work begins. This is crucial if you're indoors most of the week.

If you can't get outside, get sun through a window and crack it for fresh air if possible.

While working, resist the temptation to over-snack until lunch. Mindless snacking is an anxious habit, and eating too much crappy food will hinder your work performance and ability to be present.

This is where bringing prepared snacks is key if the offered fare is unhealthy.

Match your input to your output—if you're not moving much, don't eat too much.

Master the art of self-care in small windows:

After the work thing, take a moment to unplug. Get air and sunshine if it's light out. Hit the gym or walk/run if you didn't get exercise in the morning. Even a 15-minute speed session helps—your psyche and sociability will thank you for the reprieve.

Jetlag:

Once I arrive, it's time to take the shoes off and get my feet in the grass. If in an urban area, I'll search for a nearby park.

If I can't do that, look for a pool and swim. Grounding or immersing the body in nature does wonders to reduce inflammation.

Bonus points if I can make a workout happen right off the plane—sweating helps regulate time zone changes and improves sleep (if not landing too late).While a full gym or food prep session can sometimes be fit in, there are often smaller opportunities available to access well-being when we look for them.

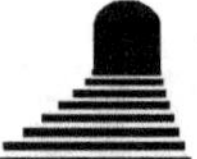

BOTTOM LINE:

- A little forethought goes a long way in planning a trip that keeps your health on track and keeps you in the groove upon return.

- Visit **www.eattheapplebook.com** for a downloadable travel checklist guide.

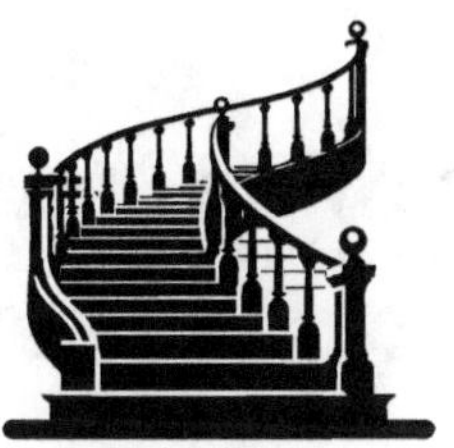

CONCLUSION

> # Do the thing, and you shall have the power.
>
> - Ralph Waldo Emerson

I have this weird expectation that if I read the right book or take another coaching program, the information will magically fix my blind spots and shortcomings.

I'll know enough, my problems will be solved, and all will be complete as I ride off into the proverbial sunset.

Perhaps not surprisingly, that never happens on its own.

"Knowing something doesn't make a damn difference," my coach, Jerry, would say. "Changing something in your life requires a clear, conscious interruption of your current patterns."

It is my hope that, in reading this book, you're seeing an access to something beyond "knowing" what to do—and now feel a sense of inspired action to do it.

To weave wellness into your version of an "impossible" schedule, whatever that looks like.

Stretching and getting some sunshine before the kids wake up... eating a piece of fruit... optimizing a commute or work trip... remembering your accomplishments and celebrating them in the moment and at a future date.

This way, we embody health and wellbeing during the brief moments between obligations and deadlines, until they just become... a part of you.

Then it becomes easier.

The phase transition is the tricky part. Phase transitions are the times during new habit development when the practices we're trying to germinate easily go out of existence. If they don't take hold with cultivation, one is left doing and thinking the same patterns (and having the same outcomes) that they did before.

Another chance to take the stairs avoided... another moldy piece of fruit thrown away... another chance at peace and gratitude in a given moment squandered.

No, what I've learned after 15+ years in health transformation is that our only way to capture and hold onto change is to be it every day. There's nowhere to "get to"—only the unfolding of results that come naturally from our habits.

Strength and energy are the outcome of increased movement.

Fat loss is the outcome of healthier food choices.

Better sleep is the outcome of conscious days and relaxing evenings.

And with your CHO schedule in hand, you can start to write your own playbook and run the scripted plays until you embody their steps and know them by heart.

There will be breakdowns and mishaps—count on it.

And the earnest attempt to get better, healthier, happier every day all but guarantees your success.

Life is a long game.

Show up big for yourself every day—just like you do for your family, your career, and everything that matters most to you.

I'm cheering for you.

Derek

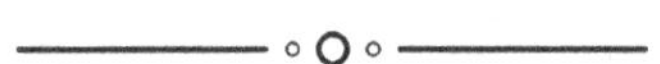

Derek Opperman is a health coach living in the 'burbs of Los Angeles. He's got two kids and a wife who inspired this book by taking up a lot of his time (in the best way!).

You can check out his podcast and learn more ways to weave wellness into your impossible schedule at **www.lifeuphealthcoaching.com**.

Got a company? You can check out what he does with companies and their employees at **www.lifeupcorporatewellness.com**.

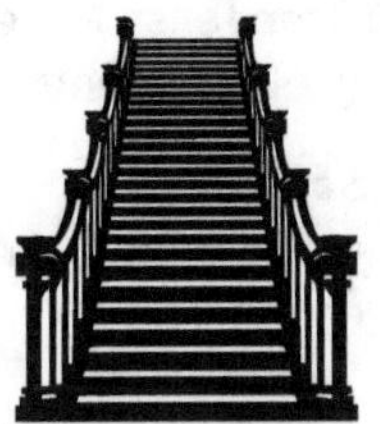

ACKNOWLEDGMENTS

My wife Joslyn for being my partner on this journey. We started out at 100 miles per hour, hardly knowing each other yet being a "yes" to starting a family together. Far from easy, yet each challenge faced has only brought us closer together. To the moon and back, my love.

Splendid and spectacular Sophie, who made me a man and a father before I thought I was ready to be. You made parenting as easy as I could've hoped, my wonderful girl.

Caius, my little bambino. You taught me good things are always worth working for. I couldn't have imagined a better son to complete our family.

Mo and David, for always believing in me. It means the world to have parents who've got my back. You were the foundation I needed to become a father who shows up unconditionally, just like you did. May you both live to be 100!

Chris Collins, for your leadership, guidance, and generosity in writing this book. What a gift to have found a book mentor standing 15 feet away from me at the gym!

Dr. Stephen Cabral, who taught me that health is so much more than calorie counting, sets, and reps. Thank you for your stand of health for all in the world, starting at home.

Sean Croxton, whose voice on *Quote of the Day Show* I listen to every morning, inspiring greatness one 15-minute podcast at a time. Your work got me up and going through more than I could possibly share. Little by little, brother.

My friends and clients who contributed their time, voice and stories to this book—Allyson, Eddie, Kristen, Shorty, Regan, Meg, Michael, Max, Andy, Sean, Jerry, Josh, Mark, and all of those unnamed here who overcame or taught me something worth sharing with the world.

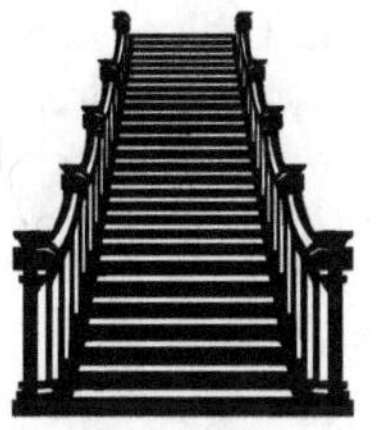

BIOGRAPHY

Derek Opperman is a 15-time-certified trainer and health coach, Fortune 500 speaker, and wellness program designer who helps busy parents and professionals rediscover how to feel lean, strong, and healthy again—just like they did before kids and career got in the way. With over 15 years of experience coaching clients, Derek blends science-backed strategies with real-life practicality, making wellness doable even for the busiest people.

His work has taken him from keynotes to kitchen tables, helping individuals and companies alike build healthier habits that last. These days, he splits his time between Boston and Los Angeles, designing health coaching programs, speaking at events, and supporting clients on their journeys.

When he's not working or doing health-related things, you can usually find him chasing his kids around the house or tackling that never-ending pile of laundry—because even coaches live in the real world.

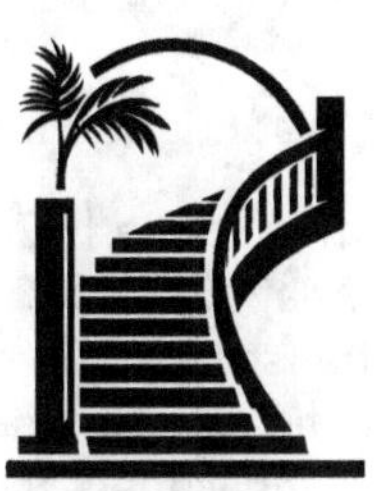

NOTES

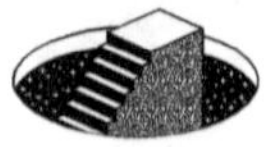

First Flight

1. Non-exercise activity thermogenesis (NEAT) includes all physical activities outside of sleeping, eating, and structured exercise—from walking to work and doing household chores to fidgeting. Physical activity-related energy expenditure accounts for 15-30% of total daily energy expenditure. For most individuals in modern society, formal exercise is negligible, meaning NEAT comprises nearly all of their activity-related calorie burn.

2. Bruce Lipton, Ph.D., is a cell biologist and pioneer in the field of epigenetics—the study of how environmental factors influence gene expression. His research demonstrated that cells respond to environmental signals rather than being controlled solely by their genetic code, challenging the concept of genetic determinism.

3. In this study, 56 participants were offered both apple slices and buttered popcorn in a competitive food environment. Despite rating the popcorn as more preferred, participants consumed significantly more of whichever food was placed within arm's reach (30cm) versus 2 meters away. The proximity effect occurred regardless of preference, demonstrating that food placement can override taste preferences in determining consumption.

4. Cardiovascular: Dancing reduces cardiovascular mortality risk (10-year follow-up, American Journal of Preventive Medicine 2016), effects equal to or better than walking. Zumba improves cardiovascular fitness and lowers resting heart rate after 12 weeks. Singing improves microvascular function in older adults with coronary artery disease (Medical College of Wisconsin 2024), heart rate patterns resemble light exercise.

Respiratory: Dance improves breathing capacity in chronic respiratory disease patients. Singing improves lung function in COPD/asthma patients, strengthens respiratory muscles (12-week RCT showed improved respiratory muscle strength).

Mental health: Meta-analysis (218 trials, 14,000+ people) found dance more effective than other exercise for reducing depression. Systematic reviews show dancing reduces depression, anxiety, stress. UCLA study: 98% reported improved mood, 96% with anxiety/depression reported benefits. Choir singing significantly reduced anxiety (p=0.013) and improved well-being (p=0.011) in 24-week study of cancer carers.

Mechanisms: Social engagement, music synchronization, expressive movement, flow states, oxytocin/endorphin release, autonomic nervous system regulation.

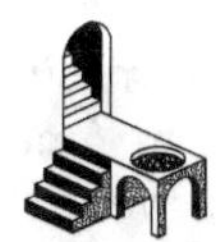

Second Flight

1. Buffey et al. (2022). Meta-analysis of 7 studies found 2-5 min walking reduced postprandial glucose by 17.01% compared to prolonged sitting.

2. Media claims of 75% of Americans chronically dehydrated lack scientific support. Actual data: 17-28% of older adults (meta-analysis: 24% of non-hospitalized elderly). Older adults most affected due to decreased thirst, medications, mobility. General adults: 25-35% consume inadequate water. Body composition: ~60% water (males 60%, females 50-55%). Brain/kidneys: 80-85% water, lungs 80-83%, heart 75-79%, bones 20-31%.

3. CDC (2022). Only 10% of adults meet vegetable recommendations and 12.3% meet fruit recommendations based on 2019 data.

4. Davis et al. (2004). University of Texas study comparing USDA data from 1950 vs. 1999 found 6-38% decline in protein, calcium, phosphorus, iron, riboflavin, and vitamin C across 43 crops.

5. Organ water percentages vary significantly. Skin: 64-75% (epidermis 60-70%, dermis 70-90%). Brain: 73-85%. Muscles: 76-79%. Lungs: 80-83%. Heart: 73-79%. Kidneys: 79-85%. Bones: 20-31%. Teeth: 8-10% (tooth enamel is the hardest substance in the human body, harder than bone). High water content essential for organ function—brain and kidneys highest, bones and teeth lowest due to mineralized composition (hydroxyapatite crystals).

6. Study of 259 bottles (11 brands, 9 countries) found microplastic contamination in 93% of bottled water. Average: 325 particles per liter, with one bottle exceeding 10,000 particles/liter. 2024 study using advanced imaging found average ~240,000 plastic particles per liter

(90% nanoplastics <1μm, 10% microplastics). Common polymers: polypropylene, polyethylene (from caps), PET (from bottles), nylon (from filtration). Nanoplastics small enough to pass through cell membranes, potentially accumulating in organs. Found in human blood, lungs, placenta, arterial plaque. Health effects poorly understood, no regulatory thresholds exist. Multiple studies show bottled water more contaminated than tap water.

7. National Human Activity Pattern Survey (NHAPS): EPA-sponsored study (1992-1994, n=9,386) found Americans spend 87% of time in enclosed buildings, 5.5-6% in vehicles, 7% outdoors. Total: 93% indoors/vehicles. Breakdown: residences 69%, office/factory 5%, other indoor locations 13%. Study conducted via 24-hour retrospective telephone diaries across 48 contiguous states. Researchers concluded time indoors has "remained fairly uniform over previous several decades." NHAPS remains most widely cited study on topic; no comprehensive update available. Canadian studies show similar patterns. EPA motivation: indoor pollutant concentrations often 2-5x higher than outdoor; understanding time-location patterns essential for exposure modeling.

8. Vitamin D benefits: Essential for bone density and calcium homeostasis; reduces fracture risk when combined with calcium (700-800 IU daily). Modulates innate and adaptive immune responses via vitamin D receptors on immune cells; deficiency linked to increased autoimmunity and infection susceptibility. Mood effects: systematic review showed efficacy for depression in studies without biological flaws; vitamin D modulates hypothalamic-pituitary-adrenal axis, regulating neurotransmitter production.

Sun exposure timing: Peak UVB for vitamin D production occurs midday (10 AM-2 PM). Recommended exposure: 5-30 minutes midday, several times weekly, depending on skin type and UV index. Light skin (types I-II): <10 minutes; medium (III-IV): <15 minutes; dark (V-VI): <30 minutes or longer. Dark skin requires 2.5x more UV exposure than light skin. Global study: maintenance of vitamin D with <15 min exposure viable only ±30° latitude. Beyond 30 min, no additional vitamin D produced; excess raises sunburn/cancer risk.

9. EPA's Total Exposure Assessment Methodology (TEAM) studies found levels of common organic pollutants 2-5 times higher inside homes than outside, regardless of rural or industrial location. EPA reports indoor pollutant levels "occasionally more than 100 times" higher than outdoor; during activities like paint stripping, levels may reach 1,000 times background outdoor levels. Sources: outgassing from pressed wood/furniture (formaldehyde, VOCs), cleaning products/aerosol sprays, pesticides, building materials, combustion (stoves, fireplaces). Inadequate ventilation causes pollutant accumulation; energy-efficient buildings without proper ventilation particularly affected. EPA ranked indoor air pollution among top 5 environmental risks to public health. Children are especially vulnerable due to higher minute ventilation and activity levels.

10. Grounding/earthing: direct skin contact with Earth's surface. Approximately 20 peer-reviewed studies suggest potential benefits. Sleep: small studies (n=12-60) report subjective improvements; 2004 study showed normalized cortisol rhythms. HRV: 2011 study (n=28) showed positive trend in heart rate variability after 40 minutes grounding, indicating parasympathetic activation. Inflammation: infrared imaging documented reduced inflammation; claims of reduced C-reactive protein (CRP) widely cited but specific peer-reviewed CRP data unclear. Other documented effects: reduced blood viscosity, accelerated wound healing, reduced pain, normalized cortisol. Limitations: small sample sizes, short durations, limited independent replication, most research by affiliated group, commercial interests present. Promising early evidence requiring larger controlled trials.

11. "Sitting is the new smoking" originated with Dr. James Levine (Mayo Clinic). Prolonged sitting (8+ hours) linked to 16% higher all-cause mortality, 34% higher cardiovascular mortality, nearly doubled type 2 diabetes risk. However, American Journal of Public Health (2018) analysis found smoking's mortality risk ~10x worse than sitting (2000+ vs. 190 excess deaths per 100,000 persons/year), concluding direct comparison "not recommended." Regular physical activity (60-75 min daily) can offset sitting effects. Nature exposure benefits: Meta-analysis (20 trials) showed forest bathing significantly reduced blood pressure vs. urban environments; 30+ min weekly in greenspace could reduce high BP prevalence by 9%. Attention Restoration Theory: natural environments restore depleted attention. Meta-analysis (12 experiments) showed working memory improved significantly more after nature vs. urban exposure. Systematic review (140+ studies, 290+ million people) documented greenspace reduces stress, improves attention, working memory, sustained focus—even after brief exposure (5-10 min).

12. Statistics on sedentary jobs from Church et al. (2011); average

American steps from Tudor-Locke & Bassett (2004); hunter-gatherer activity levels from Raichlen et al. (2017); overweight and obesity rates from Stierman et al. (2021).

13. Physical activity decline from Pontzer et al. (2012) and Raichlen et al. (2017); digestive health effects from Virtue Health (2020); circulation effects from Cleveland Clinic (2025); posture impacts from Cleveland Clinic (2025); mood and cognition impacts from meta-analyses by Huang et al. (2020) and Kandola et al. (2021); vitamin D associations from Manoy et al. (2019).

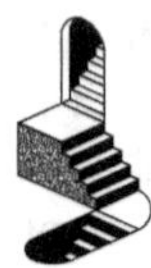

Third Flight

1. Tech neck biomechanics from Hansraj (2014); disc pressure increases from sitting posture documented by North Lakes Pain Consultants (2025); back pain economic burden from Katz (2006).

2. Research shows that slouching while seated increases lumbar disc pressure by up to 60% compared to proper upright posture. This sustained pressure contributes to disc degeneration, herniation, and chronic pain. Back pain—to which poor posture is a major contributor—costs Americans over $100 billion annually, with two-thirds of these costs attributed to lost wages and reduced productivity rather than direct medical expenses.

3. Fluorescent lighting with low-frequency flicker (100Hz from conventional ballasts) significantly increases headaches and eye strain; double-blind study showed incidence more than halved under high-frequency lighting (32kHz). Office workers under fluorescent lighting had 2x more headache episodes than natural lighting. Symptoms include ocular discomfort, burning eyes, photophobia, headaches. American Journal of Public Health (2011) study found fluorescent lighting may increase UV-related eye diseases by up to 12% due to UV emissions (290-295nm wavelengths); estimated 3,000 additional cataract cases annually in Australia. However, this study was critiqued as "too light on the science." Safe lighting range to minimize UV damage: 2000-3500K, >500 nanometers. LED cataract research limited to extreme-condition animal studies not applicable to everyday exposure. Poor lighting causes compensatory postures (leaning forward/backward) leading to neck strain and musculoskeletal problems. Color Rendering Index (CRI): measures color accuracy. CRI 80-90 considered good, 90+ excellent. Above 80, differences <10 difficult to perceive. Color temperature: 2700-3000K (warm white) reduces eye strain, promotes relaxation; 3500-4000K neutral; 5000K+ cool/daylight increases strain. High-frequency electronic ballasts reduce flicker-related symptoms.

4. Children's fruit and vegetable consumption from 2021 National Survey of Children's Health, Hamner et al. (2023).

5. Bayer (2020). In June 2020, Bayer agreed to pay $10+ billion to settle approximately 125,000 Roundup lawsuits alleging glyphosate caused cancer, following IARC's 2015 classification of glyphosate as "probably carcinogenic to humans."

6. The SCN functions as the master circadian pacemaker controlling sleep-wake timing. Darkness triggers the SCN to stimulate melatonin production via the pineal gland, which inhibits circadian arousal and promotes sleep (Saper et al., 2005).

7. White noise is defined as a random signal with equal intensity across various frequencies. This creates the characteristic "hissing" sound that can mask disruptive environmental noises and help promote sleep.

8. Americans spend approximately 87% of their time indoors and another 5.5% inside vehicles, meaning we spend about 93% of our lives in enclosed spaces. This lack of outdoor exposure affects circadian rhythm regulation, vitamin D production, and overall health.

9. Research on electromagnetic fields (EMF) and melatonin production shows highly inconsistent results. Studies examining power-frequency (50-60Hz) EMF effects on melatonin synthesis have found suppression, no effect, and even small increases. One rat study (1000 milligauss for 1 month) found marginally significant melatonin increase (opposite direction), with little effect on sleep architecture. Analysis of 100+ human/animal studies noted "significance of disruption" but results remain contradictory. Mechanisms proposed include pineal gland sensing EMF as light, but this remains "unsolved." Electromagnetic hypersensitivity (EHS): systematic review (46 double-blind experiments, 1,175 self-diagnosed EHS individuals) found no robust evidence that EMF exposure causes symptoms. EHS individuals cannot detect EMF exposure more accurately than controls. When blinded, participants reported symptoms equally with sham and real exposures, indicating nocebo effect. WHO does not recognize EHS as medical diagnosis; no diagnostic criteria or clinical practice guidelines exist. Symptoms real but not caused by EMF. Blue light from screens: well-documented to suppress melatonin production far more effectively than EMF, delaying circadian rhythms and prolonging sleep latency. 2020 meta-analysis concluded real-world WiFi levels unlikely to cause significant sleep disruptions, though high-dose RF exposure in lab settings can alter brain activity.

10. The 68% stress reduction statistic comes from "Galaxy Stress Research" conducted by cognitive neuropsychologist Dr. David Lewis at Mindlab International, University of Sussex (2009). Study involved 16 volunteers (keen readers, average age 34) using heart rate sensors and skin conductance measurements during alternating stress production/reduction activities. Results: reading for 6 minutes reduced stress by 68%, compared to listening to music (61%), drinking tea/coffee (54%), taking a walk (42%), and playing video games (21%). Important caveat: this was consultancy research that was never peer-reviewed or published in an academic journal, only reported in media outlets. Sample size small and participants self-selected as readers, limiting generalizability. Research methods expert noted findings "could serve as basis for preliminary pilot study leading to much larger-scale research study." Despite limitations, the stress-reducing benefits of reading are supported by broader research. Recent peer-reviewed studies confirm reading's positive effects on mental health: 2024 study in American Journal of Health Behavior found reading alleviates work stress and enhances job satisfaction. Reading engages imagination, requires concentration, slows heart rate, eases muscle tension, and provides "cognitive escape" from anxious thoughts—an active form of meditation where mind focuses on single engaging task.

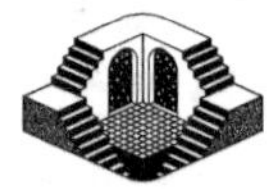

Fourth Flight

1. A University of Michigan study published in Public Health Nutrition found that adults who cook dinner at home seven or more times per week scored 3.57 points higher on the Healthy Eating Index-2015 compared to those cooking 0-2 times weekly. The Healthy Eating Index is a USDA measure of diet quality based on adherence to Dietary Guidelines for Americans.

2. At least 61 different names for sugar appear on food labels. Common examples include: Agave nectar, Barbados sugar, Barley malt, Barley malt syrup, Beet sugar, Brown sugar, Buttered syrup, Cane juice, Cane juice crystals, Cane sugar, Caramel, Carob syrup, Castor sugar, Coconut palm sugar, Coconut sugar, Confectioner's sugar, Corn sweetener, Corn syrup, Corn syrup solids, Date sugar, Dehydrated cane juice, Demerara sugar, Dextrin, Dextrose, Evaporated cane juice, Free-flowing brown sugars, Fructose, Fruit juice, Fruit juice concentrate, Glucose, Glucose solids, Golden sugar, Golden syrup, Grape sugar, High-Fructose Corn Syrup (HFCS), Honey, Icing sugar, Invert sugar, Malt syrup, Maltodextrin, Maltol, Maltose, Mannose, Maple syrup, Molasses, Muscovado, Palm sugar, Panocha, Powdered sugar, Raw sugar, Refiner's syrup, Rice syrup, Saccharose, Sorghum, Sorghum syrup, Sucrose, Sugar (granulated), Sweet sorghum, Syrup, Treacle, Turbinado sugar, Yellow sugar. Ingredients ending in "-ose" are typically forms of sugar. Manufacturers use multiple sugar names to make total sugar content less obvious - using several different sugar sources allows each to be listed separately lower on ingredient lists (which are ordered by weight), even when total sugar content is high.

3. Studies cited by FDA link these dyes to allergic reactions, hyperactivity in children, and potential carcinogenicity at high doses (FDA, 2023).

4. FDA 2023 rulemaking process. The ban phases out these additives in packaged foods, dietary supplements, and beverages, affecting over 10,000 products nationwide (noahchemicals.com).

5. Eating within 2-3 hours of bedtime negatively affects sleep quality. Study of 793 young adults found eating within 3 hours of bedtime associated with 61% increased odds of nocturnal awakenings (OR=1.61, 95% CI=1.15-2.27), though not with sleep onset latency or duration. American Time Use Survey (124,239 participants) found eating/drinking <1 hour before bed associated with 2.0-2.6x higher risk of wake after sleep onset (WASO >30 min), a key insomnia symptom. While those who ate close to bedtime slept 25-35 minutes longer, sleep was less efficient due to increased awakenings. As interval between eating and bedtime expanded, odds of WASO decreased. Mechanisms include GERD/acid reflux (stomach contents pressing against esophageal sphincter when lying down), postprandial discomfort, and reduced digestive efficiency at night due to circadian rhythms. Sleep experts recommend finishing last meal 2-4 hours before bedtime. Diet-Induced Thermogenesis (DIT): energy expenditure above basal metabolic rate for digesting, absorbing, metabolizing, and storing food. For mixed diet at energy balance, DIT = 5-15% of daily energy expenditure (typically ~10%). Thermic effect varies by macronutrient: protein 20-30%, carbohydrates 5-10%, fats 0-3%, alcohol 10-30%. Protein's high thermic effect means ~30 of every 100 protein calories used for digestion. DIT represents smallest component of total daily energy expenditure (basal metabolic rate largest, physical activity second, DIT third).

6. Ayurvedic tradition teaches that digestive capacity peaks during midday, approximately 10 AM-2 PM, making this the optimal time for the day's largest meal. This concept aligns with modern circadian rhythm research showing metabolic function, glucose tolerance, and insulin sensitivity are optimized earlier in the day. Multiple studies confirm earlier meal timing improves metabolic outcomes: same meal at 8 AM produces superior response compared to 8 PM. Research supports "eat like a king in morning, prince at noon, peasant at dinner" approach—consuming larger meals at breakfast/lunch versus dinner associated with better glucose control, insulin sensitivity, and weight management. Diet-induced thermogenesis higher in morning. Consuming most calories at dinner linked to increased obesity and metabolic syndrome risk. Though Ayurvedic philosophy and modern endocrinology arrive via different frameworks, both converge on practical recommendation: align larger meals with earlier daylight hours for optimal health.

7. The European Union has banned or restricted more than 1,600 chemicals from personal care products, while the FDA prohibits or restricts just nine ingredients for safety reasons: bithionol, mercury compounds, vinyl chloride, halogenated salicylanilides, zirconium complexes in aerosol cosmetics, chloroform, methylene chloride, chlorofluorocarbon propellants, and hexachlorophene. Japan and other countries also maintain strict cosmetic ingredient regulations

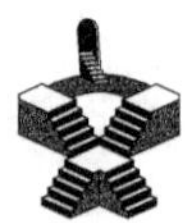

Fifth Flight

1. Health experts generally recommend finishing meals 2-4 hours before bedtime to allow adequate digestion time. Eating too close to sleep can cause acid reflux, indigestion, and disrupted sleep quality. The thermic effect of food (TEF)—the energy required to digest, absorb, and process nutrients—typically accounts for about 10-15% of total daily caloric expenditure, though this varies by macronutrient composition.

2. National GI Survey (2018) of 71,812 Americans found 61% reported experiencing ⩾1 gastrointestinal symptom in the past week, with nearly two-thirds of surveyed individuals burdened by digestive symptoms. Most commonly reported: heartburn/reflux (30.9%), abdominal pain (24.8%), bloating (20.6%), diarrhea (20.2%), and constipation (19.7%). Females, younger individuals, non-Hispanic whites, higher-educated individuals, and those with medical comorbidities more likely to report symptoms. Important distinction: while 60-70 million Americans have diagnosed digestive diseases (18-21% of population), symptom prevalence far exceeds formal diagnoses since less than 20% of individuals with GI symptoms consult healthcare providers. Claims-based prevalence of diagnosed digestive diseases (2019): 24.2% among Medicaid beneficiaries, 33.2% among private insurance enrollees, 51.5% among Medicare beneficiaries. Digestive disease burden substantial and rising in United States.

3. Research by Valter Longo, director of the University of Southern California's Longevity Institute, demonstrated that a 5-day fasting-mimicking diet (FMD)—providing around 600 calories on day 1, then approximately 300 calories on days 2-5—can yield nearly all the benefits of water-only fasting while maintaining high compliance rates. Clinical trials showed the FMD reduced biological age by an average of 2.5 years, improved cardiovascular markers including blood pressure and cholesterol, decreased abdominal and liver fat, reduced insulin resistance and HbA1c levels, and activated cellular repair mechanisms including stem cell regeneration. The diet had a 91.8% compliance rate across studies, with fatigue as the most common side effect. Multiple randomized controlled trials have confirmed these metabolic and anti-aging benefits, making FMD a more tolerable alternative to complete fasting while delivering comparable physiological effects.

4. According to the U.S. Census Bureau's 2019 American Community Survey, the average one-way commute time in the United States reached an all-time high of 27.6 minutes, translating to 55.2 minutes roundtrip daily. This represents a 27% increase since 1980, when the average was 21.7 minutes one-way. Over a standard work year (250 days), this amounts to approximately 230 hours—nearly 10 full days—spent commuting annually. Commute times vary significantly by location: New York has the longest average at 33.4 minutes one-way, while South Dakota has the shortest at 16.6 minutes. Major cities see even longer commutes, with NYC averaging 34.7-40.7 minutes one-way.

The COVID-19 pandemic temporarily reduced commute times as remote work became prevalent, with 2021 seeing one-way commutes drop to 25.6 minutes (51.2 minutes roundtrip). However, as return-to-office mandates increased, 2022 data showed commutes rising back to 26.4 minutes one-way (52.8 minutes roundtrip), continuing to approach pre-pandemic levels. Mode of transportation significantly affects travel time: bus commuters average 46.6 minutes one-way, while those driving alone average 25.5 minutes.

Research consistently shows longer commutes negatively impact physical and mental health. Extended commuting is associated with increased stress, anxiety, elevated cortisol levels, reduced sleep quality, less time for physical activity, and higher rates of obesity and cardiovascular problems. Traffic congestion imposes additional stress through unpredictability and loss of control. Economic impacts are substantial: Americans lose over $1,500 per driver annually due to congestion-related delays and fuel costs. For parents, long commutes reduce family time and limit participation in children's activities, making proximity to work an important consideration for family wellbeing.

5. According to the U.S. Census Bureau's 2024 American Community Survey, approximately 86.7% of American workers commute to work, meaning they leave home to travel to a workplace rather than working from home. The remaining 13.3% work from home—a figure that has remained elevated since the COVID-19 pandemic but is declining from the 17.9% peak in 2021. Pre-pandemic (2019), only 5.7% of workers worked from home.

Among commuters, the vast majority drive. In 2024, 69.2% of workers drove alone to work, with an additional ~9% carpooling, bringing total automobile commuting to approximately 78% of all workers. Only 3.7% use public transportation, while roughly 4% walk, bike, or use other means. The dominance of driving has remained remarkably stable: in 2019, 75.9% drove alone; by 2022 it dropped to 68.7% and has held steady at 69.2% in 2023-2024.

Commute time represents a significant daily time investment that many people leave unoptimized. With an average roundtrip of 55 minutes daily, this represents nearly 230 hours annually—time that could be used for audiobooks, podcasts, language learning, phone calls with family, or simply decompressing. Research shows that how people use their commute time affects their stress levels and job satisfaction. Some treat it as "me time" for mental preparation or relaxation, while others experience it as wasted time and stress. For parents, commute time often means less time with children and reduced participation in family activities, making intentional use of that time especially important.

6. High-intensity interval training (HIIT) can produce cardiovascular and metabolic adaptations similar to traditional moderate-intensity exercise but in about 40% less time. During these intense bursts, your body recruits Type II muscle fibers, ramps up ATP production up to 100-fold, and triggers mitochondrial adaptations that improve how efficiently your cells use energy. HIIT is particularly effective for reducing visceral fat, improving insulin sensitivity, and building cardiovascular capacity. However, for pure strength and muscle gains, traditional resistance training remains king—HIIT isn't a replacement for lifting weights. The real sweet spot? Combining both approaches in your routine.

7. Sleep research began mid-19th century; major breakthrough occurred 1953 with discovery of REM sleep. Sleep medicine established as medical field in 1970s (first sleep lab 1970, American Academy of Sleep Medicine founded 1975). Classic rat experiments demonstrated total sleep deprivation resulted in death within 2-3 weeks due to sepsis, revealing sleep's critical role in immune function. Early epidemiological studies (1970s-1980s, >1 million subjects) showed mortality rates significantly increased with <4 hours or >10 hours sleep nightly. Research exploded past two decades: peer-reviewed sleep journals tripled since 2005. Modern studies link inadequate sleep to hypertension, obesity, diabetes, cardiovascular disease, neurodegeneration, accelerated aging, and DNA damage. Sleep facilitates memory consolidation, cognitive performance, emotional regulation, and metabolic homeostasis. Brain clears waste via glymphatic system during sleep.

8. Cortisol secretion follows a 24-hour circadian rhythm, with peak levels occurring around 7-8am in the morning (the active phase) and lowest secretion around 2-4am at night. Additionally, the cortisol awakening response (CAR) causes cortisol levels to increase by 38-75% within 30-45 minutes after waking, independent of the underlying circadian rhythm. This morning surge helps prepare the body for daily activities. While some sources suggest delaying coffee consumption until after cortisol peaks (around 9:30-11am) to optimize caffeine's effectiveness, no studies have demonstrated superior energizing effects with delayed morning coffee compared to immediate consumption. Individual factors such as stomach sensitivity, anxiety levels, and caffeine tolerance may be more important than timing.

9. Caffeine has a half-life of 3-7 hours in most adults (average ~5 hours), meaning that half of the caffeine consumed remains in the body after this time. The stimulating effects typically last 3-5 hours, though caffeine can disrupt sleep even when consumed 6-8 hours before bedtime. A 2023 systematic review found that to avoid reductions in total sleep time, coffee should be consumed at least 8.8 hours prior to bedtime. Caffeine increases cortisol secretion by elevating ACTH production at the pituitary gland, which in turn stimulates adrenal cortisol production. Studies show that while partial tolerance develops with regular consumption (300-600 mg/day), cortisol responses are not completely eliminated, particularly with afternoon caffeine intake.

10. Cytochrome P450 1A2 (CYP1A2) is the enzyme responsible for metabolizing 80-95% of caffeine in the body. Genetic variation in the CYP1A2 gene (particularly the rs762551 polymorphism) determines whether individuals are "fast" or "slow" caffeine metabolizers. Approximately 50% of the population carries genetic variants (AC or CC genotypes) that make them slow metabolizers, meaning caffeine remains in their system longer and has more pronounced effects on sleep, blood pressure, and anxiety. Fast metabolizers (AA genotype) clear caffeine more quickly from their systems. This genetic variation has been shown to modify the association between coffee consumption and risks of myocardial infarction, hypertension, and other health outcomes.

11. L-theanine is a non-protein amino acid found naturally in tea leaves, particularly green tea and matcha. Research shows that L-theanine (200-400 mg doses) can reduce stress and anxiety by influencing neurotransmitters including GABA, dopamine, and serotonin, and by promoting alpha brain wave activity associated with relaxation. Multiple studies have demonstrated that when combined with caffeine, L-theanine can improve cognitive performance and alertness while reducing the jittery side effects of caffeine. Green tea naturally contains both caffeine (20-50 mg per cup) and L-theanine (6-50 mg per cup), with the optimal ratio for stress-reducing effects occurring when the molar ratio of caffeine to L-theanine is less than 2-3. The combination provides smooth, sustained energy without the anxiety or jitteriness that caffeine alone can produce.

12. The thermic effect of food (TEF), also called diet-induced thermogenesis, is the energy required for digestion, absorption, and processing of nutrients. TEF accounts for approximately 10% of total daily energy expenditure in healthy adults consuming a mixed diet, though it can range from 8-15% depending on diet composition. For example, if someone expends 2,000 calories per day, approximately 200 calories are used for digestion. The thermic effect varies significantly by macronutrient: protein has the highest TEF at 20-30% (meaning 20-30% of protein calories are burned during digestion), carbohydrates have a moderate TEF of 5-15%, and fats have the lowest TEF at 0-5%. This is why high-protein diets can have a slight metabolic advantage and why protein keeps people feeling fuller longer. However, for an overall balanced diet containing all three macronutrients, the total thermic effect averages around 10% of daily caloric intake, not the 30% that applies only to protein digestion specifically.

13. Delta-9-tetrahydrocannabinol (THC) is the primary psychoactive compound in cannabis that produces the "high" associated with marijuana use. Research consistently shows that THC suppresses REM (Rapid Eye Movement) sleep, the stage of sleep critical for memory consolidation, emotional processing, and learning. Studies demonstrate that THC use decreases the percentage of time spent in REM sleep and increases REM latency (the time it takes to enter REM sleep). A 2008 systematic review found that while THC increases deep slow-wave sleep, it simultaneously reduces REM sleep, disrupting the delicate balance of sleep architecture. Chronic cannabis users show significantly decreased REM sleep percentage (as low as 17.7% compared to the normal 20-25%) and increased REM latency (averaging 114.5 minutes). This is why many cannabis users report having fewer dreams or no dream recall. When heavy users stop THC consumption, they often experience "REM rebound"—intense, vivid dreams as the brain attempts to recover lost REM sleep. Sleep disturbances during cannabis withdrawal are reported by 67-73% of adults and can persist for 6-7 weeks. While THC's REM suppression has been explored therapeutically for PTSD-related nightmares and certain sleep disorders, chronic REM suppression in healthy individuals can impair cognitive function, memory formation, and emotional regulation—all critical functions that occur during this "brain-supporting" stage of sleep.

Final Flight

1. Gus Turner, "Michael Phelps Reveals His Mythic 12,000-Calorie Diet 'Is Not Real,'" Men's Health, June 15, 2017

2. Wim Hof is a Dutch extreme athlete known for cold tolerance feats. In 2007, he climbed to 7,200-7,400 meters on Mount Everest wearing only shorts and shoes before stopping due to foot injury—he didn't summit. He's set over 26 world records and teaches the "Wim Hof Method" combining cold therapy, breathing, and meditation.

On metabolism: Cold exposure increases energy expenditure through shivering thermogenesis (muscle contractions generating heat) and non-shivering thermogenesis (brown adipose tissue burning fat). Mild cold (16-19°C) raises metabolic rate ~5%; intense cold with shivering can double it temporarily. Brown adipose tissue accounts for 120-370 kcal/day when active, representing 15-25% of resting energy expenditure. However, these increases occur during exposure and fade quickly after. The body compensates by increasing appetite. A sustained 15%+ metabolic boost from cold exposure hasn't been established in controlled studies.

3. Cold exposure has two faces. When nasal temperature drops by 5°C—what happens breathing cold air—immune function in your nose drops nearly 50%. The nose produces extracellular vesicles (EVs) that neutralize viruses, but cold reduces EV production by 42%. This explains winter's infection spike.

Deliberate cold exposure triggers different effects. Cold water immersion increases norepinephrine 2-3 fold and epinephrine 1.5 fold, mobilizing white blood cells from the spleen into circulation. Studies show increased lymphocytes and natural killer cells immediately after exposure. The lymphatic system also contracts, temporarily boosting circulation.

The catch: norepinephrine both mobilizes immune cells and suppresses their function. Long-term studies of winter swimmers show modest increases in activated T cells after 6 weeks, though researchers note effects are "slight" with "biological significance yet to be elucidated." Think hormesis—controlled stress training adaptive responses. Not a cure-all, but potentially helpful for those who tolerate it well.

4. Cold exposure spikes noradrenaline 2-5x and dopamine 250%. Cold receptors in the skin send electrical impulses to the brain, activating the sympathetic nervous system and releasing beta-endorphins. This creates immediate alertness and arousal.

5. T5. The depression hypothesis comes from a 2008 Medical Hypotheses paper—a journal that publishes speculative ideas, not proven treatments. Later case studies showed promise (a 2018 BMJ report found cold water swimming helped one woman's depression), but large trials are lacking.

The catch: a 2021 systematic review found cold exposure impaired cognition in 15 of 18 studies. Executive function, working memory, attention, and processing speed all decline during cold exposure, with impairments persisting 60+ minutes after rewarming—even once body temperature normalizes. The trade-off is real: enhanced mood and alertness at the cost of temporary cognitive performance. Not ideal right before tasks requiring sharp thinking.

6. The global dietary supplements market has experienced explosive growth over the past two decades, driven by increasing health consciousness, aging populations, and a shift toward preventive healthcare. The market was valued at approximately $152 billion in 2021 and grew to $192.65 billion by 2024. Multiple research firms project continued strong growth, with estimates ranging from $300-414 billion by 2033, representing a compound annual growth rate (CAGR) of 6.4-8.9% depending on the source and market segments included.

The U.S. represents the largest single-country market, valued at approximately $64 billion in 2024 and projected to reach $103-162 billion by 2033. Growth rates vary by category: vitamins hold the largest market share at 28-40%, followed by herbal supplements at 32%, and protein/sports nutrition. Specific segments show even higher growth—prenatal supplements are growing at 11-13% CAGR, weight management at 14% CAGR, and online sales at 10-13% CAGR as e-commerce becomes increasingly dominant.

The COVID-19 pandemic significantly accelerated supplement adoption, with sales increasing 50% between 2018 and 2020 as consumers focused on immune support. Consumer demographics are shifting: adults remain the largest user group (63-64% of market), but the geriatric population and infant/children segments are growing fastest.

Distribution has evolved from primarily specialty stores to widespread availability through pharmacies, mass retailers, and online platforms, with over-the-counter sales representing 75-76% of the market.

7. The 2015-2020 Dietary Guidelines for Americans recommend "nutritional needs should be met primarily through foods" rather than supplements. Whole foods contain the "food matrix"—fiber, phytonutrients, and micronutrients working synergistically to enhance absorption. An orange provides vitamin C plus fiber, calcium, and protein; a supplement provides only isolated ascorbic acid.

Meta-analyses show multivitamin supplementation doesn't prevent disease or premature death in well-nourished populations. Current guidelines recommend supplements only for specific circumstances: diagnosed deficiencies, pregnancy/breastfeeding, aging adults with decreased absorption, certain medications (like metformin depleting B12), and limited sun exposure requiring vitamin D. Harvard Health advises improving diet before using supplements. Taking supplements to mask poor eating habits has proven ineffective and may create false nutritional security.

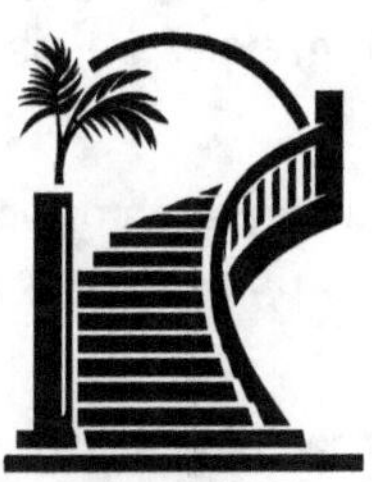

REFERENCES

Agency for Toxic Substances and Disease Registry. (2015). *Taking an exposure history: What are possible sources of indoor air pollution.* https://www.atsdr.cdc.gov/csem/exposure-history/Indoor-Air-Pollution-Sources.html

Allison, K. C., et al. (2020). Circadian rhythms and meal timing: impact on energy balance and body weight. *Current Opinion in Biotechnology*, 70, 1-6.

Almario, C. V., et al. (2018). Burden of gastrointestinal symptoms in the United States: Results of a nationally representative survey of over 71,000 Americans. *American Journal of Gastroenterology*, 113(11), 1701-1710.

Anglin, R. E., Samaan, Z., Walter, S. D., & McDonald, S. D. (2013). Vitamin D deficiency and depression in adults: systematic review and meta-analysis. *British Journal of Psychiatry*, 202(2), 100-107.

Angarita, G. A., Emadi, N., Hodges, S., & Morgan, P. T. (2016). Sleep abnormalities associated with alcohol, cannabis, cocaine, and opiate use: A comprehensive review. *Addiction Science & Clinical Practice*, *11*(1), 9.

Aranow, C. (2011). Vitamin D and the immune system. *Journal of Investigative Medicine*, 59(6), 881-886.

Armstrong, L. E., Bergeron, M. F., Muñoz, C. X., & Kavouras, S. A. (2024). Low daily water intake profile—is it a contributor to disease? *Sage Open Medicine*, 12.

Babson, K. A., Sottile, J., & Morabito, D. (2017). Cannabis, cannabinoids, and sleep: A review of the literature. *Current Psychiatry Reports*, *19*(4), 23.

Bailey, R. L., Gahche, J. J., Miller, P. E., Thomas, P. R., & Dwyer, J. T. (2013). Why US adults use dietary supplements. *JAMA Internal Medicine*, *173*(5), 355-361.

Baranwal, N., et al. (2023). Sleep physiology, pathophysiology, and sleep hygiene. Progress in Cardiovascular Diseases, 77, 59-69.

Bierman, A., & Rea, M. S. (2012). Climate change, fluorescent lighting, and eye disease: A little too light on the science [Letter to the editor]. *American Journal of Public Health*, *102*(8), e6.

Bolla, K. I., Lesage, S. R., Gamaldo, C. E., Neubauer, D. N., Funderburk, F. R., Cadet, J. L., David, P. M., Verdejo-Garcia, A., & Benbrook, A. R. (2008).

Sleep disturbance in heavy marijuana users. *Sleep, 31*(6), 901-908.

Brandhorst, S., & Levine, M. E. (2024). Fasting-mimicking diet causes hepatic and blood markers changes indicating reduced biological age and disease risk. *Nature Communications, 15*, 1309.

Buffey, A. J., Herring, M. P., Langley, C. K., Donnelly, A. E., & Carson, B. P. (2022). The acute effects of interrupting prolonged sitting time in adults with standing and light-intensity walking on biomarkers of cardiometabolic health in adults: A systematic review and meta-analysis. *Sports Medicine, 52*(8), 1765-1787.

Calcagno, M., Kahleova, H., Alwarith, J., Burgess, N. N., Flores, R. A., Busta, M. L., & Barnard, N. D. (2019). The thermic effect of food: A review. *Journal of the American College of Nutrition, 38*(6), 547-551.

Cannon, B., & Nedergaard, J. (2004). Brown adipose tissue: Function and physiological significance. Physiological Reviews, 84(1), 277-359.

Centers for Disease Control and Prevention. (2022). Adults meeting fruit and vegetable intake recommendations — United States, 2019. *Morbidity and Mortality Weekly Report, 71*(1), 1-9.

Chen, K. Y., Brychta, R. J., Linderman, J. D., Smith, S., Courville, A., Dieckmann, W., Herscovitch, P., Millo, C. M., Remaley, A., Lee, P., & Celi, F. S. (2013). Brown fat activation mediates cold-induced thermogenesis in adult humans in response to a mild decrease in ambient temperature. Journal of Clinical Endocrinology & Metabolism, 98(7), E1218-E1223.

Chondronikola, M., Volpi, E., Børsheim, E., Porter, C., Annamalai, P., Enerbäck, S., Lidell, M. E., Saraf, M. K., Labbe, S. M., Hurren, N. M., Yfanti, C., Chao, T., Andersen, C. R., Cesani, F., Hawkins, H., & Sidossis, L. S. (2014). Brown adipose tissue improves whole-body glucose homeostasis and insulin sensitivity in humans. Diabetes, 63(12), 4089-4099.

Church, T. S., Thomas, D. M., Tudor-Locke, C., Katzmarzyk, P. T., Earnest, C. P., Rodarte, R. Q., Martin, C. K., Blair, S. N., & Bouchard, C. (2011). Trends over 5 decades in U.S. occupation-related physical activity and their associations with obesity. *PLoS ONE, 6*(5), e19657.

Clift, S., et al. (2017). Singing and chronic obstructive pulmonary disease: A randomized controlled trial. *BMJ Open,* 7(1), e014151.

Cornelis, M. C., El-Sohemy, A., Kabagambe, E. K., & Campos, H. (2006). Coffee, CYP1A2 genotype, and risk of myocardial infarction. *JAMA, 295*(10), 1135-1141.

Crispim, C. A., et al. (2019). *British Journal of Nutrition.*

Davis, D. R., Epp, M. D., & Riordan, H. D. (2004). Changes in USDA food composition data for 43 garden crops, 1950 to 1999. *Journal of the American College of Nutrition, 23*(6), 669-682.

Dodd, F. L., Kennedy, D. O., Riby, L. M., & Haskell-Ramsay, C. F. (2015). A double-blind, placebo-controlled study evaluating the effects of caffeine and L-theanine both alone and in combination on cerebral blood flow, cognition and mood. *Psychopharmacology, 232*(14), 2563-2576.

Environmental Working Group. (2022, October 26). Personal care product chemicals banned in Europe but still found in U.S. https://www.ewg.org/news-insights/news/2022/10/personal-care-product-chemicals-banned-europe-still-found-us

Falla, M., Micarelli, A., Hüfner, K., Pavei, G., Bonato, M., Bisschoff, C. A., ... & Schena, F. (2021). The effect of cold exposure on cognitive performance in healthy adults: A systematic review. *International Journal of Environmental Research and Public Health, 18*(18), 9725.

Fancourt, D., et al. (2019). Psychosocial singing interventions for the mental health and well-being of family carers of patients with cancer: Results from a longitudinal controlled study. *BMJ Open,* 9(8), e026995.

Gardiner, C., Weakley, J., Burke, L. M., Roach, G. D., Sargent, C., Maniar, N., Townshend, A., & Halson, S. L. (2023). The effect of caffeine on subsequent sleep: A systematic review and meta-analysis. *Sleep Medicine Reviews, 69,* 101764.

Gates, P. J., Albertella, L., & Copeland, J. (2014). The effects of cannabinoid administration on sleep: A systematic review of human studies. *Sleep Medicine Reviews, 18*(6), 477-487.

Gibala, M. J., et al. (2021). Evidence-based effects of high-intensity interval training on exercise capacity and health. International Journal of Environmental Research and Public Health, 18(13), 7201.

Girard, O. (2022). *The posture manual: Your guide to a pain-free life.* https://oliviergirard.ch/en/boutique/the-posture-manual/

Hamner, H. C., Dooyema, C. A., Blanck, H. M., Kompaniyets, L., & Lansford, K. (2023). Fruit, vegetable, and sugar-sweetened beverage intake among young children, by state — United States, 2021. Morbidity and Mortality Weekly Report, 72(7), 165-170.

Hansraj, K. K. (2014). Assessment of stresses in the cervical spine caused by posture and position of the head. *Surgical Technology International, 25*, 277-279.

Harvard Health Publishing. (2015). Get nutrients from food, not supplements. *Harvard Health Letter.* Harvard Medical School. Retrieved from https://www.health.harvard.edu/press_releases/get-nutrients-from-food-not-supplements

Hooper, L., Bunn, D. K., Abdelhamid, A., et al. (2023). Low-intake dehydration prevalence in non-hospitalised older adults: Systematic review and meta-analysis. *Age and Ageing,* 52(7), afad101.

Huang, Y., Li, L., Gan, Y., Wang, C., Jiang, H., Cao, S., & Lu, Z. (2020). Sedentary behaviors and risk of depression: A meta-analysis of prospective studies. *Translational Psychiatry, 10*(1), 26. _

Iao, S. I., et al. (2021). Associations between bedtime eating or drinking, sleep duration and wake after sleep onset. *British Journal of Nutrition,* 127(12), 1888-1900.

Ideno, Y., et al. (2017). Blood pressure-lowering effect of Shinrin-yoku (forest bathing): A systematic review and meta-analysis. *BMC Complementary and Alternative Medicine, 17,* 409.

Kandola, A., del Pozo Cruz, B., Osborn, D. P. J., Stubbs, B., Choi, K. W., & Hayes, J. F. (2021). Impact of replacing sedentary behaviour with other movement behaviours on depression and anxiety symptoms: A prospective cohort study in the UK Biobank. *BMC Medicine, 19*(1), 133. _

Katz, J. N. (2006). Lumbar disc disorders and low-back pain: Socioeconomic factors and consequences. *Journal of Bone and Joint Surgery, 88*(Suppl 2), 21-24. _

Kesner, A. J., & Lovinger, D. M. (2020). Cannabinoids, endocannabinoids and sleep. *Frontiers in Molecular Neuroscience, 13,* 125. _

Klepeis, N. E., Nelson, W. C., Ott, W. R., Robinson, J. P., Tsang, A. M., Switzer, P., Behar, J. V., Hern, S. C., & Engelmann, W. H. (2001). The National Human Activity Pattern Survey (NHAPS): A resource for assessing exposure to environmental pollutants. *Journal of Exposure Analysis and Environmental Epidemiology, 11*(3), 231-252.

Krishnan, S., & Cooper, J. A. (2014). Effect of dietary fatty acid composition on substrate utilization and body weight maintenance in humans. *European Journal of Nutrition, 53*(3), 691-710. _

Kulinski, J. P., et al. (2024). Effects of singing on vascular health in older adults with coronary artery disease: A randomized, crossover trial. *Frontiers in Cardiovascular Medicine*, 11, 1345858.

Langan, A. (2018). Getting nutrients in food vs supplementation. Parkview Health. Retrieved from https://www.parkview.com/blog/getting-nutrients-in-food-vs-supplementation

Lee-Kwan, S. H., Moore, L. V., Blanck, H. M., Harris, D. M., & Galuska, D. (2022). Adults meeting fruit and vegetable intake recommendations—United States, 2019. *Morbidity and Mortality Weekly Report*, *71*(1), 1-9.

Lewis, D. (2009). *Galaxy stress research*. Mindlab International, Sussex University, UK. [Unpublished consultancy report]

Lipton, B. H. (2015). *The Biology of Belief: Unleashing the power of consciousness, matter & miracles* (10th anniversary ed.). Hay House.

Liu, P., Han, Y., Li, W., & Zhao, S. (2024). Psychological effects of reading on alleviating work stress and enhancing job satisfaction: An analytical study. *American Journal of Health Behavior*, *48*(2), 425-437.

Longo, V. D., & Mattson, M. P. (2014). Fasting: Molecular mechanisms and clinical applications. *Cell Metabolism*, *19*(2), 181-192.

Lovallo, W. R., Whitsett, T. L., al'Absi, M., Sung, B. H., Vincent, A. S., & Wilson, M. F. (2005). Caffeine stimulation of cortisol secretion across the waking hours in relation to caffeine intake levels. *Psychosomatic Medicine*, *67*(5), 734-739.

Lucas, R. M., Neale, R. E., Madronich, S., McKenzie, R. L. (2024). Globally estimated UVB exposure times required to maintain sufficiency in vitamin D levels. *Nutrients*, 16(10), 1489.

Manoy, P., Yuktanandana, P., Tanavalee, A., Anomasiri, W., Ngarmukos, S., Tanpowpong, T., & Honsawek, S. (2017). Vitamin D supplementation improves quality of life and physical performance in osteoarthritis patients. *Nutrients, 9*(8), 799.

Marlatt, K. L., & Ravussin, E. (2017). Brown adipose tissue: An update on recent findings. Current Obesity Reports, 6(4), 389-396.

Mason, S. A., Welch, V. G., & Neratko, J. (2018). Synthetic polymer contamination in bottled water. *Frontiers in Chemistry*, 6, 407.

McCann, D., Barrett, A., Cooper, A., et al. (2007). Food additives and hyperactive behaviour in 3-year-old and 8/9-year-old children in the community: a randomised, double-blinded, placebo-controlled trial. *The Lancet*, 370(9598), 1560-1567. U.S. Food and Drug Administration. (2023). *FDA assessment of artificial food dyes: Health effects and regulatory action*. Retrieved from fda.gov

Mensink, G. B., Fletcher, R., Gurinovic, M., Huybrechts, I., Lafay, L., Serra-Majem, L., ... & Stephen, A. M. (2013). Mapping low intake of micronutrients across Europe. *British Journal of Nutrition*, *110*(4), 755-773.

Merom, D., Ding, D., Stamatakis, E. (2016). Dancing participation and cardiovascular disease mortality: A pooled analysis of 11 population-based British cohorts. *American Journal of Preventive Medicine*, 50(6), 756-760.

Mitchell, H. H., Hamilton, T. S., Steggerda, F. R., & Bean, H. W. (1945). The chemical composition of the adult human body and its bearing on the biochemistry of growth. *Journal of Biological Chemistry*, 158(3), 625-637.

Moan, J., Porojnicu, A. C., & Dahlback, A. (2008). At what time should one go out in the sun? *Advances in Experimental Medicine and Biology*, 624, 86-88.

Moore, L. V., & Thompson, F. E. (2015). Adults meeting fruit and vegetable intake recommendations—United States, 2013. *Morbidity and Mortality Weekly Report*, *64*(26), 709-713.

Muller, M. D., Kim, C. H., Bellar, D. M., Ryan, E. J., Seo, Y., Gunstad, J., & Glickman, E. L. (2012). Acute cold exposure and cognitive function: Evidence for sustained impairment. *Ergonomics*, *55*(7), 792-798.

Murrock, C. J., & Graor, C. H. (2023). Evidence of the effects of dance interventions on adults mental health: A systematic review. *American Journal of Health Behavior*, 47(4), 602-616.

National Institute of Diabetes and Digestive and Kidney Diseases. (2025). Digestive diseases statistics for the United States.

National Public Radio. (2020, June 24). Bayer to pay more than $10 billion to resolve cancer lawsuits over weedkiller Roundup. https://www.npr.org/2020/06/24/882949098/bayer-to-pay-more-than-10-billion-to-resolve-roundup-cancer-lawsuits

North Lakes Pain Consultants. (2025, April 14). How poor posture can lead to chronic spine pain. https://northlakespain.com/how-poor-posture-can-lead-to-lead-to-chronic-spine-pain/

O'Callaghan, F., Muurlink, O., & Reid, N. (2018). Effects of caffeine on sleep quality and daytime functioning. *Risk Management and Healthcare Policy, 11*, 263-271.

Peters, B., et al. (2024). Meal timing and its role in obesity and associated diseases. *Frontiers in Endocrinology*, 15, 1359772.

Pontzer, H., Raichlen, D. A., Wood, B. M., Mabulla, A. Z., Racette, S. B., & Marlowe, F. W. (2012). Hunter-gatherer energetics and human obesity. *PLoS ONE, 7*(7), e40503.

Privitera, G. J., & Zuraikat, F. M. (2014). Proximity of foods in a competitive food environment influences consumption of a low calorie and a high calorie food. *Appetite, 76*, 175-179.

Qian, N., Gao, X., Lang, X., et al. (2024). Rapid single-particle chemical imaging of nanoplastics by SRS microscopy. *Proceedings of the National Academy of Sciences*, 121(3), e2300582121.

Quatela, A., Callister, R., Patterson, A., & MacDonald-Wicks, L. (2016). The energy content and composition of meals consumed after an overnight fast and their effects on diet induced thermogenesis: A systematic review, meta-analyses and meta-regressions. *Nutrients, 8*(11), 670.

Raichlen, D. A., Pontzer, H., Harris, J. A., Mabulla, A. Z., Marlowe, F. W., Snodgrass, J. J., Berbesque, J. C., Raichlen, E. E., & Wood, B. M. (2017). Physical activity patterns and biomarkers of cardiovascular disease risk in hunter-gatherers. *American Journal of Human Biology, 29*(2), e22919.

Rautiainen, S., Manson, J. E., Lichtenstein, A. H., & Sesso, H. D. (2016). Dietary supplements and disease prevention—a global overview. *Nature Reviews Endocrinology, 12*(7), 407-420.

Reed, G. W., & Hill, J. O. (1996). Measuring the thermic effect of food. *The American Journal of Clinical Nutrition, 63*(2), 164-169.

Röösli, M., Dongus, S., Jalilian, H., Eyers, J., Esu, E., Oringanje, C. M., et al. (2024). The effects of radiofrequency electromagnetic fields exposure on tinnitus, migraine and non-specific symptoms in the general and working population: A systematic review and meta-analysis on human observational studies. *Environmental International, 183*, 108338.

Rubin, G. J., Das Munshi, J., & Wessely, S. (2005). Electromagnetic hypersensitivity: A systematic review of provocation studies. *Psychosomatic Medicine, 67*(2), 224-232.

Rubin, G. J., Nieto-Hernandez, R., & Wessely, S. (2010). Idiopathic environmental intolerance attributed to electromagnetic fields (formerly 'electromagnetic hypersensitivity'): An updated systematic review of provocation studies. *Bioelectromagnetics, 31*(1), 1-11.

Sabag, A., et al. (2018). The compatibility of concurrent high intensity interval training and resistance training for muscular strength and hypertrophy. Sports Medicine, 48(11), 2472-2489.

Schierenbeck, T., Riemann, D., Berger, M., & Hornyak, M. (2008). Effect of illicit recreational drugs upon sleep: Cocaine, ecstasy and marijuana. *Sleep Medicine Reviews, 12*(5), 381-389.

Shanahan, D. F., et al. (2016). Health benefits from nature experiences depend on dose. *Scientific Reports, 6*, 28551.

Shepard, J. W., et al. (2005). History of the development of sleep medicine in the United States. Journal of Clinical Sleep Medicine, 1(1), 61-82.

Shevchuk, N. A. (2008). Adapted cold shower as a potential treatment for depression. *Medical Hypotheses, 70*(5), 995-1001.

Sleep Foundation. (2024). Is it bad to eat before bed? https://www.sleepfoundation.org/nutrition/is-it-bad-to-eat-before-bed

Šrámek, P., Šimečková, M., Janský, L., Šavlíková, J., & Vybíral, S. (2000). Human physiological responses to immersion into water of different temperatures. *European Journal of Applied Physiology, 81*(5), 436-442.

Stenfors, C. U. D., et al. (2019). Positive effects of nature on cognitive performance across multiple experiments. *Frontiers in Psychology, 10*, 1413.

Stierman, B., Afful, J., Carroll, M. D., Chen, T. C., Davy, O., Fink, S., Fryar, C. D., Gu, Q., Hales, C. M., Hughes, J. P., Ostchega, Y., Storandt, R. J., & Akinbami, L. J. (2021). National Health and Nutrition Examination Survey 2017–March 2020 prepandemic data files: Development of files and prevalence estimates for selected health outcomes. *National Health Statistics Reports, 158.*

St-Onge, M. P., et al. (2016). Effects of diet on sleep quality. *Advances in Nutrition*, 7(5), 938-949.

Tudor-Locke, C., & Bassett, D. R. (2004). How many steps/day are enough? Preliminary pedometer indices for public health. *Sports*

Medicine, 34(1), 1-8.

Twohig-Bennett, C., & Jones, A. (2018). The health benefits of the great outdoors: A systematic review and meta-analysis of greenspace exposure and health outcomes. *Environmental Research, 166*, 628-637.

UCSF SugarScience. (n.d.). *Hidden in plain sight.* University of California, San Francisco. https://sugarscience.ucsf.edu/hidden-in-plain-sight/

Unalp-Arida, A., & Ruhl, C. E. (2024). Burden of digestive diseases in the United States population: Rates and trends. *American Journal of Gastroenterology, 120*(9), 1987-1997.

Unno, K., Furushima, D., Hamamoto, S., Iguchi, K., Yamada, H., Morita, A., Horie, H., & Nakamura, Y. (2018). Stress-reducing function of matcha green tea in animal experiments and clinical trials. *Nutrients, 10*(10), 1468.

U.S. Census Bureau. (2024). Census Bureau releases new brief about travel to work since pandemic's onset [Press release]. Retrieved from https://www.census.gov/newsroom/press-releases/2024/travel-to-work-since-pandemic.html

U.S. Census Bureau. (2024). *Commuting in the United States: 2022* (Report No. ACS-52). Retrieved from https://www2.census.gov/library/publications/2024/demo/acsbr-018.pdf

U.S. Census Bureau. (2024). United States commuting at a glance: American Community Survey 1-year estimates. Retrieved from https://www.census.gov/topics/employment/commuting/guidance/acs-1yr.html

U.S. Department of Agriculture & U.S. Department of Health and Human Services. (2020). *Dietary Guidelines for Americans, 2020-2025* (9th ed.). Retrieved from https://www.dietaryguidelines.gov/

U.S. Environmental Protection Agency. (2025). *The inside story: A guide to indoor air quality.* https://www.epa.gov/indoor-air-quality-iaq/inside-story-guide-indoor-air-quality

U.S. Environmental Protection Agency. (2025). *Why indoor air quality is important to schools.* https://www.epa.gov/iaq-schools/why-indoor-air-quality-important-schools

U.S. Food and Drug Administration. (2023). Rulemaking: *Phase-out of petroleum-based food dyes.* Federal Register. Noah Chemicals. (2025).

US ban on artificial dyes in food products. Retrieved from noahchemicals. com

U.S. Food and Drug Administration. (n.d.). Prohibited & restricted ingredients in cosmetics. https://www.fda.gov/cosmetics/cosmetics-laws-regulations/prohibited-restricted-ingredients-cosmetics

U.S. Department of Health and Human Services & U.S. Department of Agriculture. (2015). *2015-2020 Dietary Guidelines for Americans* (8th ed.). Retrieved from https://health.gov/dietaryguidelines/2015/guidelines/

U.S. Geological Survey. (n.d.). *The water in you: Water and the human body.* Water Science School. https://www.usgs.gov/special-topics/water-science-school/science/water-you-water-and-human-body

Vallance, J. K., et al. (2018). Evaluating the evidence on sitting, smoking, and health: Is sitting really the new smoking? *American Journal of Public Health, 108*(11), 1478-1482.

van der Lans, A. A., Hoeks, J., Brans, B., Vijgen, G. H., Visser, M. G., Vosselman, M. J., Hansen, J., Jörgensen, J. A., Wu, J., Mottaghy, F. M., Schrauwen, P., & van Marken Lichtenbelt, W. D. (2013). Cold acclimation recruits human brown fat and increases nonshivering thermogenesis. Journal of Clinical Investigation, 123(8), 3395-3403.

van der Schueren, M. A., Laviano, A., Blanchard, H., Jourdan, M., Arends, J., & Baracos, V. E. (2018). The balance between food and dietary supplements in the general population. *Proceedings of the Nutrition Society, 78*(1), 97-109.

Van Iterson, E. (2025, May 16). How a sedentary lifestyle impacts your health. Cleveland Clinic. https://health.clevelandclinic.org/sedentary-lifestyle

Van Someren, E. J. W., & Riemersma-van der Lek, R. F. (2007). Live to the rhythm, slave to the rhythm. *Sleep Medicine Reviews, 11*(6), 465-484.

van Tulleken, C., Tipton, M., Massey, H., & Harper, C. M. (2018). Open water swimming as a treatment for major depressive disorder. *BMJ Case Reports*, bcr-2018-225007.

Villablanca, P. A., Alegria, J. R., Mookadam, F., Holmes, D. R., Wright, R. S., & Levine, J. A. (2015). Nonexercise activity thermogenesis in obesity management. *Mayo Clinic Proceedings, 90*(4), 509-519.

Virtue Health. (2020). What happens to your gut in prolonged sitting and poor posture? https://www.vitruehealth.com/blog/what-happens-to-your-gut-in-prolonged-sitting-and-poor-posture

Walls, H. L., Walls, K. L., & Benke, G. (2011). Eye disease resulting from increased use of fluorescent lighting as a climate change mitigation strategy. *American Journal of Public Health, 101*(12), 2222-2225.

Webb, A. R., & Holick, M. F. (1988). The role of sunlight in the cutaneous production of vitamin D3. *Annual Review of Nutrition*, 8, 375-399.

Wei, M., Brandhorst, S., Shelehchi, M., Mirzaei, H., Cheng, C. W., Budniak, J., Groshen, S., Mack, W. J., Guen, E., Di Biase, S., Cohen, P., Morgan, T. E., Dorff, T., Hong, K., Michalsen, A., Laviano, A., & Longo, V. D. (2017). Fasting-mimicking diet and markers/risk factors for aging, diabetes, cancer, and cardiovascular disease. *Science Translational Medicine, 9*(377), eaai8700.

Westerterp, K. R. (2004). Diet induced thermogenesis. *Nutrition & Metabolism, 1*(1), 5.

Wewege, M., et al. (2017). The effects of high-intensity interval training vs. moderate-intensity continuous training on body composition in overweight and obese adults. Obesity Reviews, 18(6), 635-646.

Wikipedia. (n.d.). White noise. Retrieved December 6, 2024, from https://en.wikipedia.org/wiki/White_noise

Wilkins, A. J., Nimmo-Smith, I., Slater, A. I., & Bedocs, L. (1989). Fluorescent lighting, headaches and eyestrain. *Lighting Research & Technology, 21*(1), 11-18.

Williams, J. L., Everett, J. M., D'Cunha, N. M., Sergi, D., Georgousopoulou, E. N., Keegan, R. J., McKune, A. J., Mellor, D. D., Anstice, N., & Naumovski, N. (2020). The effects of green tea amino acid L-theanine consumption on the ability to manage stress and anxiety levels: A systematic review. *Plant Foods for Human Nutrition, 75*(1), 12-23.

Wired for Adventure. (2022, April 19). Meet the man who climbed Everest in shorts. https://www.wiredforadventure.com/the-man-who-climbed-everest-in-shorts/

Wolfson, J. A., Leung, C. W., & Richardson, C. R. (2020). More frequent cooking at home is associated with higher Healthy Eating Index-2015 score. Public Health Nutrition, 23(13), 2384-2394.

World Health Organization. (2005). *Electromagnetic hypersensitivity.*

https://www.who.int/teams/environment-climate-change-and-health/radiation-and-health/non-ionizing/hypersensitivity

Wust, R. C., Morse, C. I., de Haan, A., Jones, D. A., & Degens, H. (2012). Effects of extremely low-frequency electromagnetic fields on melatonin and sleep. *Environmental Health: Journal of Biosocial Medicine, 5*(1), 10904.

Yahoo Finance. (2024). Commuting to work in the US: Facts and statistics. Retrieved from https://finance.yahoo.com/news/commuting-us-facts-statistics-200426818.html

Yamada, Y., Toramoto, S., Schutz, Y., Itoi, A., Ikegami, S., Maeda, Y., ... & Yoshida, T. (2021). Influence of cold exposure on energy expenditure in humans: Consensus, controversies, and future perspectives. *Journal of Circumpolar Health, 80*(1), 1886235.

Yoneshiro, T., Aita, S., Matsushita, M., Kayahara, T., Kameya, T., Kawai, Y., Iwanaga, T., & Saito, M. (2013). Recruited brown adipose tissue as an antiobesity agent in humans. Journal of Clinical Investigation, 123(8), 3404-3408.

Zhou, S. F., Yang, L. P., Zhou, Z. W., Liu, Y. H., & Chan, E. (2009). Insights into the substrate specificity, inhibitors, regulation, and polymorphisms and the clinical impact of human cytochrome P450 1A2. *The AAPS Journal, 11*(3), 481-494.

NOTES

NOTES

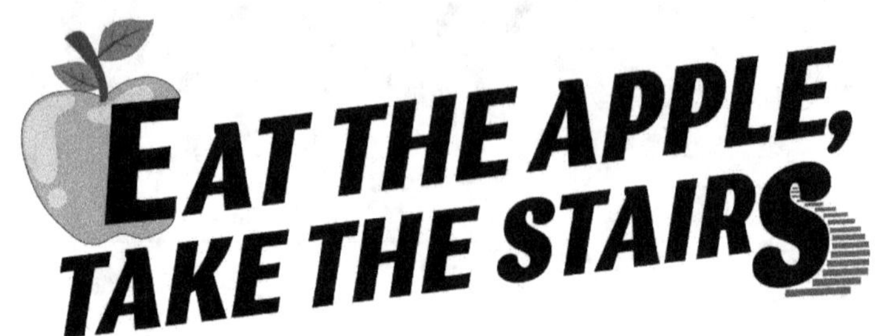

WEAVING WELLNESS THROUGH YOUR "IMPOSSIBLE" SCHEDULE

BY DEREK OPPERMAN

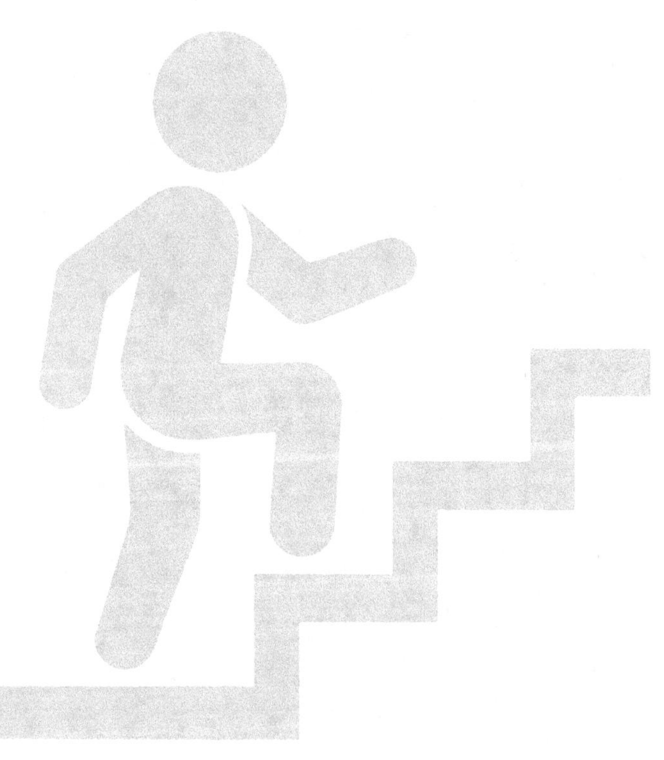

www.ingramcontent.com/pod-product-compliance
Lightning Source LLC
Chambersburg PA
CBHW051734250726

48659CB00001B/59